KETO DESSERTS
COOKBOOK

The 40 Simplest and Fasty Recipes for Weight Loss

Jessica Logan

Table of Contents

INTRODUCTION 5

PRESS THE RESET BUTTON OF YOUR DIGESTIVE SYSTEM

HAVE YOUR ENERGY LEVELS TAKEN A NOSEDIVE? 7
SO, WHAT CHANGED? 7
IT STARTS WITH THE FOOD YOU EAT **8**
EVER-INCREASING STRESS LEVELS **8**
YOUR METABOLISM DEBUNKED! **9**
WHY IS MY METABOLISM SLOW? **10**

A LIGHTBULB MOMENT!

ENTER THE KETO DIET! **11**
LET'S START AT THE VERY BEGINNING **12**
HOW DO I KNOW THAT KETO WILL WORK FOR ME? **12**
THE LIFESTYLE **13**

40 SIMPLEST AND FASTY

KETO DESSERTS 15

*Sugar-Free Mint Ice Cream **15***
*Keto Avocado & Prosciutto Fat Bombs **17***
*Homemade Keto Nutella **19***
*Lemon Cheesecake Fat Bombs **21***
*Keto Peach Cobbler **23***
*Blissful Matcha-Pistachio Balls **25***
*Cashew Butter Fat Bombs **27***
*Keto Cinnamon Roll Mousse **29***
*Keto Almond Fudge Fat Bomb **31***
*Butter Onion Bacon Dessert **33***
*Spiced Low-Carb Coconut Milk Avocado Shake **35***
*Jalapeno Popper Fat Bombs **37***
*Keto Cheese Roll-Ups **39***
*Keto Biscuits & Gravy **41***
*Low-Carb Crab Fat Bombs **43***
*Healthy Low-Carb Bagels **45***
*Keto BLT Baked Avocado Eggs **47***
*Keto Parmesan Croutons **51***

Low-Carb Italian Flaxseed Bread Crackers **53**
Low-Carb Pina Colada Fat Bombs **55**
Keto Lemon Poppy Seed Muffins Recipe **57**
Low-Carb Garlic Chia Bread Crackers **59**
Low-Carb Bread Twists **61**
Simple and Quick Keto Muffins **63**
Chocolate & Pumpkin Protein Pudding **65**
Cauliflower Breakfast Pizza **67**
Tasty Keto Drop Biscuits **69**
Chocolate Protein Fudge **71**
Lime & Coconut Avocado Popsicles **73**
Soft Rosemary-Infused Bagels **75**
Fluffy Turmeric Veggie Buns **77**
Almond Flour Italian Crackers **79**
Chocolate Peanut Butter Milkshake **81**
Cheese & Fruit-Stuffed Panini **83**
Healthy Grain-Free Bagels **85**
Superfood Keto Shake **87**
Healthy Mocha Ice Bombs **89**

IN SUMMARY... 91

CONCLUSION 92

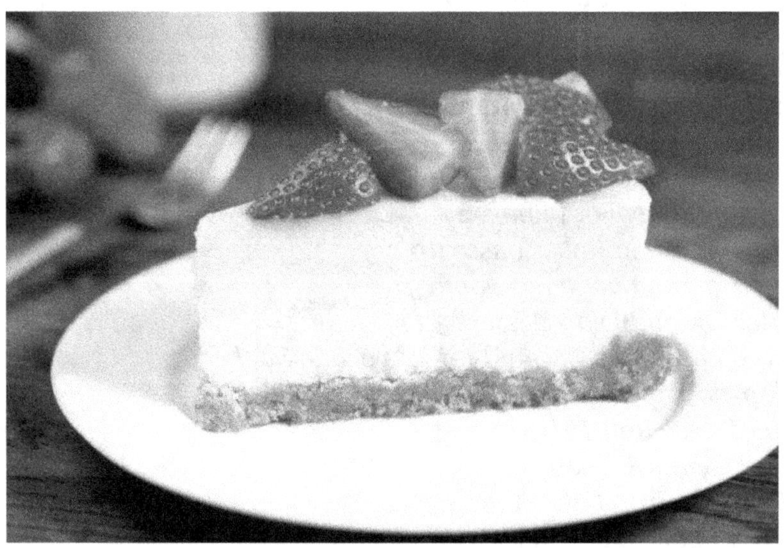

Introduction

Ever had a guilty pleasure that is deemed to be not so healthy, but no matter how much you try shaking it off, you can't bring yourself to stay away from it? For me, desserts are my guilty pleasure. If my memory serves me well, my mom said since I was two, I have been dreaming of what my dessert for dinner would be the moment I wake up.

You can almost tell that this habit led to a love-hate relationship with food and weight loss. There were times where I would go without a single taste of dessert for a whole week (trust me, this is an eternity for me!) then on the eighth day I would hear a moist chocolate cake with a scoop of ice cream calling out my name, and when I couldn't take it anymore, I would bury my head in a humongous piece of cake and an entire tub of ice cream to make up for the seven days I went without dessert.

It took three years of this unhealthy habit for me to finally admit to myself that I needed help, and this was the beginning of my self-education that started with me researching online and consulting with nutritionists. The more I learned, the more I fell in love with the world of nutrition, and this led to me pursuing a degree in fitness and nutrition.

Remember my love for desserts? This motivated me to learn how to create tasty recipes, but that was not going directly to my waistline. As you will see in the desserts in the recipe section, I use natural and healthy ingredients that, instead of storing fat in your body, promote the burning of fat in your body.

My inspiration for this book comes from my lifelong love story with desserts. Other than that, when I was starting out on the self-education journey, I wanted to see if other people were struggling with the same problem I was struggling with and lo and behold, there was a whole world of people struggling with eating their favorite foods and losing weight!

So, what can you expect in this book?

One, the tastiest desserts you are ever going to taste! Two, a great world of nutritional knowledge that teaches you how your body receives food and how you can train your body to crave healthy foods. And last, how to finally lose weight after all the struggles you've been through trying to shed those extra pounds.

Without further ado, let's get to it!

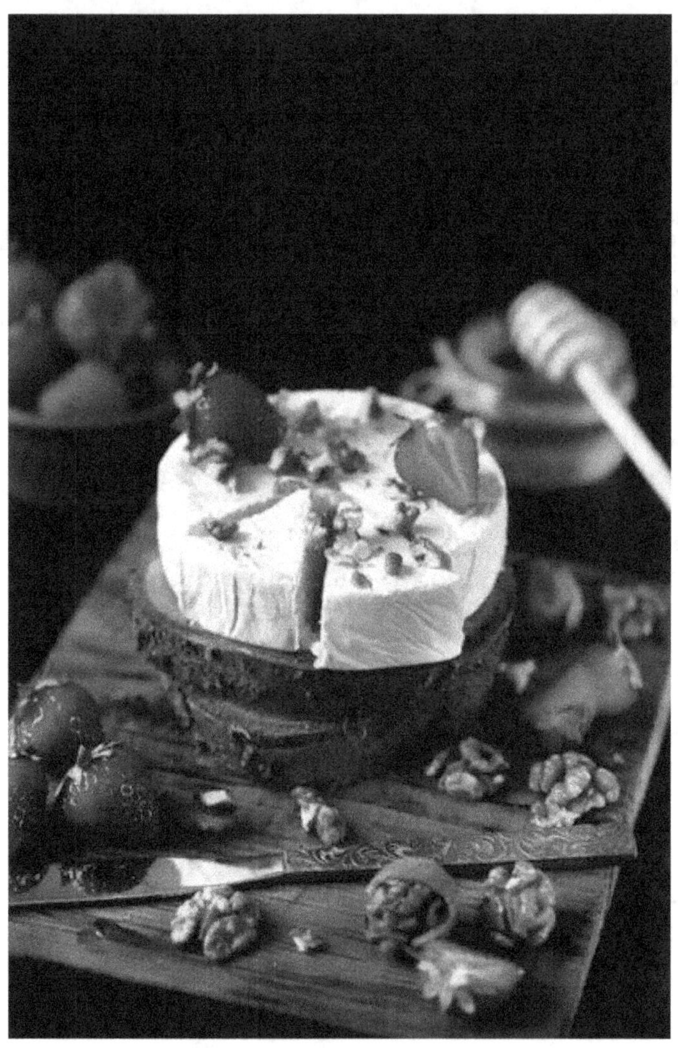

Press the Reset Button of Your Digestive System

Food, as we know it today, has undergone one of the most rapid metamorphosis processes from naturally grown foods to over-refined and processed foods that have been stripped of most of their nutrition, if not all! As a result, your digestive system has found itself in a precarious position where it is expected to digest the food you eat and provide your body with energy, but it hasn't got a clue on how to deal with processed sugars, cholesterol, and sodium-laden foods.

It is no wonder then that we are in a constant battle with obesity, diabetes, cancer, and high blood pressure, among other chronic illnesses.

Have your energy levels taken a nosedive?

I remember when I was at the center of the toughest tug-of-war between my love for dessert and my desire to lose weight, my energy levels were almost non-existent, and I relied on about six cups of coffee and sugar-laden foods to take me through the day.

It's crazy how many of us take energy for granted until we start experiencing chronic fatigue even right after waking up. Energy is the prime indicator of vitality—the very essence of what it means to be alive. Before I embarked on a self-healing journey, the last time I truly remembered firing on all cylinders was when I was a kid. The energizer bunny had nothing on me!

So, what changed?

What caused the sudden shift from the mental clarity and sharpness that gave you the confidence that you could do anything that you set out to do to the heavy cloud that hangs over your head from the moment you wake up?

Well, you could say that as a kid, you didn't have to think about how you were going to pay your bills, your rent, feed your kids, etc. While the fact that life is challenging as an adult and there's nothing much we can do about that, it is not meant to be impossible.

I will tell you one thing: The chronic fatigue you have been experiencing is your body's way of crying out for help, and we are going to look at exactly how this happens.

It starts with the food you eat

In this age of instant everything, it is safe to say that health has been thrown out the window as convenience has been welcomed through the front door. Natural food as we know it is highly perishable, so what could the food industry do to keep food on the shelves longer? Get rid of all aspects of food that make it go bad, meaning strip it of all its nutrients. Without nutrients, the food would taste bland, so replace the nutrients with artificial ingredients and taste enhancers that will never go bad and help whatever nutrients were left to stay longer. We are talking about preservatives, additives, artificial sugars, and fats.

What this means for us consumers is we are eating dead food as all living aspects of food were destroyed. If we borrow a saying from the world of computers, "garbage in garbage out," we are then dead men and women walking!

Our bodies were designed to feed from Mother Nature, and eating all these over-processed foods heavily compromises our digestive system, and it starts sending out signals to you that could be in the form of an upset stomach and dwindling energy levels. If not addressed, this then leads to more serious conditions developing, such as kidney disease, liver disease, digestive problems, diabetes, and more.

Ever-increasing stress levels

Most of us are familiar with the fight-or-flight response from our bodies when faced with a potentially dangerous situation. This is a primal instinct that is meant to keep you safe and is usually triggered in specific situations that your brain deems to be harmful. However, today's lifestyle is such that we are continually exposed to stress. So you can imagine, your body responds to each stressful situation with the fight-or-flight response. Eventually, your body gets worn out.

Some of the fight responses involve inflammation, which can help a wound heal faster or protect you from allergenic or toxic substances or help a sprained joint heal faster by using pain to keep you from subjecting it to any weight.

When inflammation gets triggered on a near-continuous basis, the communication between your brain and your adrenal glands gets scrambled. Your adrenals secret hormones that respond to particular situations. So, when this response is now continuous, the constant ineffective communication between your brain and adrenal glands tires your brain, and this is the genesis of you experiencing unexplainable fatigue, lethargy, and cognitive decline as your brain's effort of triggering a response to increased stress is now changed into negative stress.

The fatigue you experience is from your body tirelessly trying to work to rid the stress it is registering to no avail, and the fatigue is the first signal that something is not right. If this persists, your kidneys and liver are not able to function properly, and toxins start accumulating in your body. Your liver gets so overwhelmed that it is not able to efficiently burn fat for energy, your digestive system is also not able to process the few nutrients you eat if your diet is unhealthy, your blood vessels become thinner from the clogging of fat, and the heart is unable to pump blood effectively to all your organs. This is the onset of chronic illnesses!

Phew! That was quite the lesson, but let's do one more and look at what you can do to reverse all these! Yes, it's possible to reverse all the damage!

Your metabolism debunked!

We all have that one friend who can eat a whole pizza, a whole box of donuts, or a whole tub of ice cream and not even add an ounce of weight while, on the other hand, just a sniff of cookies baking seems to expand your waistline.

I remember throwing all caution to the wind every time I ate my dessert because if I were to start thinking of what that bite of my moist chocolate cake would do to my hips and waistline, I would stop myself from eating it. Then I'd be grumpy, and after a lot of debate with my conscience, I would wake up at 2:00 am to eat the chocolate cake...and this time, not one slice, but two!

Turns out, I just had to learn about metabolism and how to rev it up! Well, here is a crash course on what metabolism is and the role it plays.

Your body is made up of very tiny energy-producing processing plants known as mitochondria. These are tasked with fueling all your body's processes by converting the food you consume and the oxygen you breathe into fuel. When we refer to metabolism, we are talking about your mitochondria. A fast metabolism, therefore, means that the body can convert food to fuel in an efficient way, and the opposite is true.

Why is my metabolism slow?

Genetics play a hand in your metabolism. For example, if you come from a family with a history of diabetes, you have a high chance of having mitochondria that are not very effective in burning food for fuel compared to the average person.

The food you eat also plays a role in determining your metabolism. Your brain reads the food you eat as pieces of coded information that it uses to send signals to your cells through your nervous system. Processed foods have a very high-calorie level that can be overwhelming for your mitochondria as it tries to convert them to energy and can actually "break the system," thus triggering inflammation that, if not addressed, leads to disease.

Starving yourself, on the other hand, slows down your metabolism. This is because your brain reads this as there being a lack of food, and as such, it has to conserve all its energy sources, and one of the ways it does this is to hoard all your fat during the short term. This explains why yo-yo dieting never works, and it only causes you to gain weight.

For the longest time, we have been wrongly conditioned to believe that weight-loss boils down to two things: reducing your food intake and exercising with the end goal being achieving calorie deficiency (using up more calories than you eat).

I say wrongly conditioned because all this approach does is create a love-hate relationship with your food and exercise because it involves deprivation. It forces you to be so hard on yourself, believing that the only way to lose weight is to have self-restraint. ***The one day you "slip" and eat a little chocolate, you look down upon yourself for not having strong willpower, and if you are overweight, you start thinking that everyone who looks at you is judging you for not having the necessary discipline to lose weight.***

While calories do matter, I am going to introduce you to one of the tastiest and enjoyable ways to a healthy body and weight loss.

Enter the keto diet!

We have so far established that every little thing we put in our mouth directly affects how our bodies function. Food is not just the grease that keeps the wheel of your body rolling, it is a unique and special means by which you can boost your health and vitality.

Every time we hear the word diet, the first thing that comes to mind is childlike food portions of super bland food. Well, I'm pleased to let you know that the keto diet is no such diet. First of all, it doesn't promise you "21 days" of solving all your weight loss problems; it is a lifestyle through and through.

Let's start at the very beginning

Have you ever tried answering why our ancestors had very healthy bodies? Why there were very few instances of chronic illnesses? That notwithstanding the lack of scientific and medical progress, they still lived longer than our current generation?

You might have already guessed the answer: They purely nourished themselves with food directly from plants and animals that were not genetically modified.

Sugar primarily came from honey, fruits, and nectar from particular plants, and the fruits back then were not scientifically modified to make them sweeter. There was no processing or refinement. They also had to do a lot of walking as modes of transportation were not as abundant as they are today. It is no wonder they were as fit as a fiddle!

How do I know that keto will work for me?

Before we answer this question, here is a brief explanation of what it is. Known as the ketogenic diet, it prescribes high-fat and low-carbohydrate foods that train your body to make fats its primary energy source as opposed to carbohydrates.

Back to the question, the keto diet is going to work for you based on the following reasons:

- *Sustainable weight loss*

A high-carbohydrate diet and not eating enough healthy fats is the primary reason for weight gain. Since your body, under normal circumstances, would choose carbs as its primary energy source, it ends up storing fat. Additionally, a high-carb diet makes your body retain a lot of water. In fact, for every one molecule of glucose, there are two molecules of water attached to it. This is the reason why you lose a lot of water weight within your first two weeks of the keto diet or any other diet that calls for reduced carbohydrate consumption.

The keto diet helps your body burn fat for fuel, and so you don't store any fat.

- *It heavily reduces blood sugar and insulin levels*

The carbohydrates you eat are converted to glucose by insulin, which is then used as fuel by your body. With the low intake of carbs in the keto diet, very little insulin is produced by your body, thus directly lowering your blood glucose levels. If you are pre-diabetic or fully diabetic, the keto diet will help reverse your symptoms.

- *Long-lasting satiation*

Fatty food generally keeps you full longer, and you can finally forget about the 10:30 am hunger pangs that happen like clockwork. You will finally be more than comfortable with only three meals, or less in a day!

- *Increased mental focus*

The keto diet has been long in use to treat children who have epilepsy and neurological disorders. The brain, when studied, has shown that it works better when ketones (fats processed in your liver) are the primary energy source and not glucose. This is because your brain is able to reserve energy when using ketones and so it doesn't have to work overtime, thus helping you stay alert and also keeping it in top fighting shape against pathogens.

The lifestyle

If you are tired of trying all the diets in the world with no success and are ready to lose weight healthily as you enjoy some of the tastiest food and desserts you are ever going to eat, then keto is for you! The one thing you need to keep in mind is that the keto diet will literally reset your metabolic system, and the first two weeks will not be easy sailing. However, speaking from my own experience, it is all worth it, and I wouldn't have it any other way! All you have to remember is every time you feel a little bit of discomfort, it is your body adjusting to not using carbohydrates for fuel to using fat.

When you reduce your carb intake, you get into something called ketosis, where your body now uses fat for energy. This is, therefore, not something you do for a week or month as every time you increase your carbohydrate intake, your body will go back to using carbohydrates for fuel. The best part about the keto diet is that it cuts out all refined foods and artificial sugars as these are the typical definition of empty calories.

This is the secret that I wanted to share with you all along. The keto diet is what restored my broken relationship with food, and you will see this in the dessert recipes I have shared with you. They are very simple, use readily available ingredients, and did I mention how mouthwateringly delicious they are?

It's now time to move on to the fun part—DESSERT!

Sugar-Free Mint Ice Cream

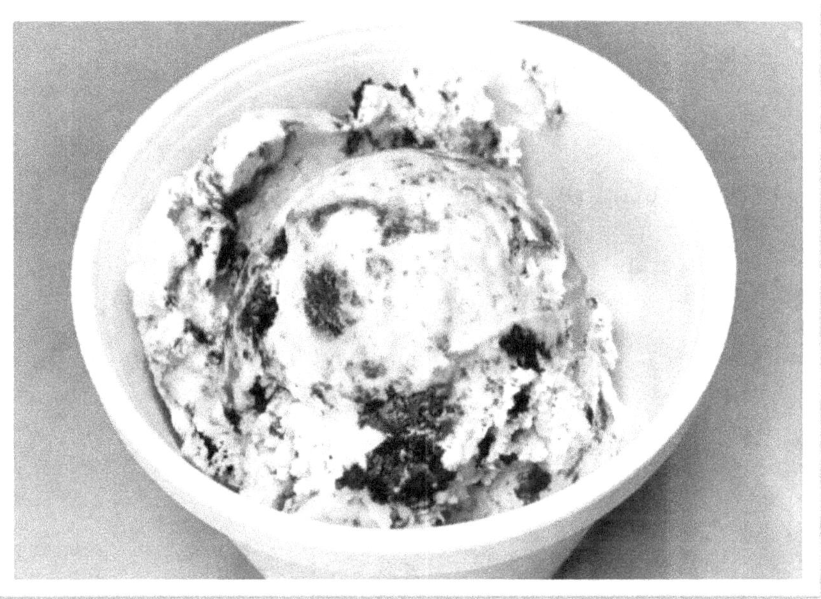

Yields: 3 servings
Total Time: 8 minutes
Prep Time: 5 minutes
Cook Time: 3 minutes

Ingredients

- ¼ cup almond milk
- 2 cups heavy whipping cream
- 4 egg yolks
- 1 teaspoon stevia powder
- ¼ teaspoon mint extract
- 3 tablespoons peppermint-flavored syrup
- 5 drops green food coloring

- In a microwave-safe bowl, combine almond milk and cream. Microwave for 2 minutes.
- In another bowl, mix the remaining ingredients and then stir into the heated cream mixture. Microwave for 1 minute and stir until well combined. Microwave again for 30 seconds and then stir. Strain the mixture into a bowl and freeze for about 30 minutes.
- Transfer to ice cream maker and follow the instructions to freeze until firm. Enjoy!

Nutritional Information per Serving
Calories: 315;
Total Fat: 35 g;
Carbs: 12 g;
Dietary Fiber: 2 g;
Sugars: 8 g;
Protein: 5 g;
Cholesterol: 0 mg;
Sodium: 13 mg

Keto Avocado & Prosciutto Fat Bombs

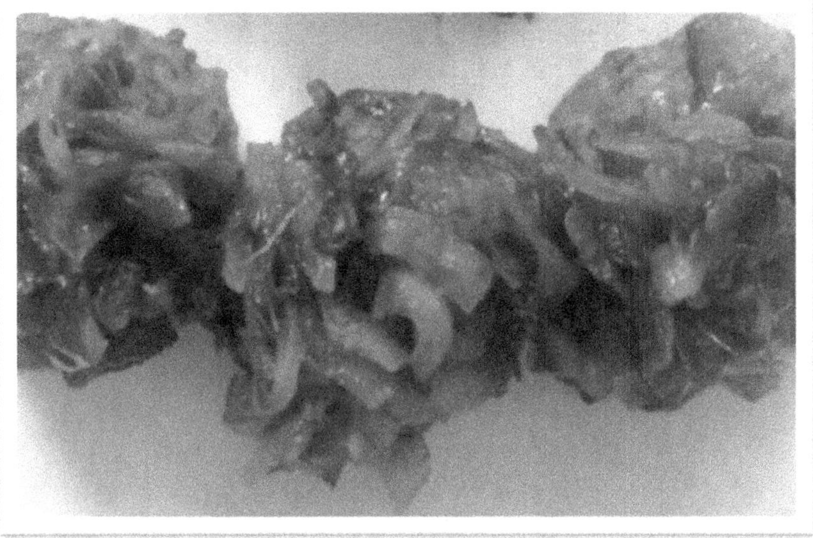

Yields: 12 Fat Bombs
Total Time: 10 minutes
Prep Time: 10 minutes
Cook Time: N/A

Ingredients

- 12 slices prosciutto

- 1 avocado, diced into 12 slices

- ½ cup freshly squeezed lemon juice

- Add avocado slices to a large bowl. Drizzle with fresh lemon juice.
- Lay the prosciutto slices on a flat work surface and top each with an avocado slice.
- Drizzle with more fresh lemon juice and roll each prosciutto up to form wraps. Enjoy!

Nutritional Information per Serving

Calories: 99;
Total Fat: 10 g;
Carbs: 2 g;
Dietary Fiber: 2 g;
Sugars: 0 g;
Protein: 3 g;
Cholesterol: 0 mg;
Sodium: 7 mg

Homemade Keto Nutella

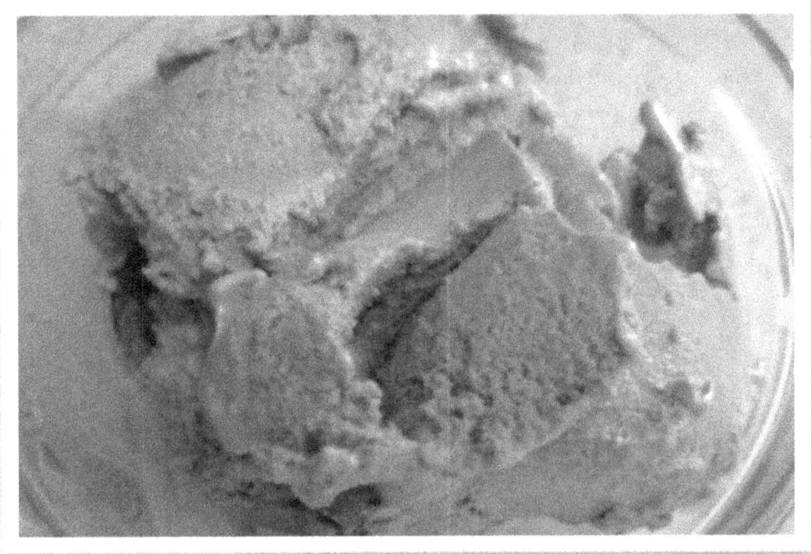

Yields: 6 servings
Total Time: 10 minutes
Prep Time: 10 minutes
Cook Time: N/A

Ingredients

- ¾ cup toasted hazelnuts
- 3 tablespoons melted coconut oil
- 2 tablespoons cocoa powder
- 3 scoops protein powder
- ½ teaspoon vanilla extract
- 2 tablespoons powdered Sweetener
- Pinch of salt

- Add hazelnuts to your food processor and grind until finely ground.
- Add in coconut oil and process the mixture into butter.
- Add in the remaining ingredients and process until creamy and smooth.
- Serve with celery or carrot sticks.

Nutritional Information per Serving

Calories: 501;
Total Fat: 33.6 g;
Carbs: 15.2 g;
Protein: 28.8 g;
Dietary Fiber: 4.6 g;
Sugars: 3.8 g;
Cholesterol: 0 mg;
Sodium: 349 mg

Lemon Cheesecake Fat Bombs

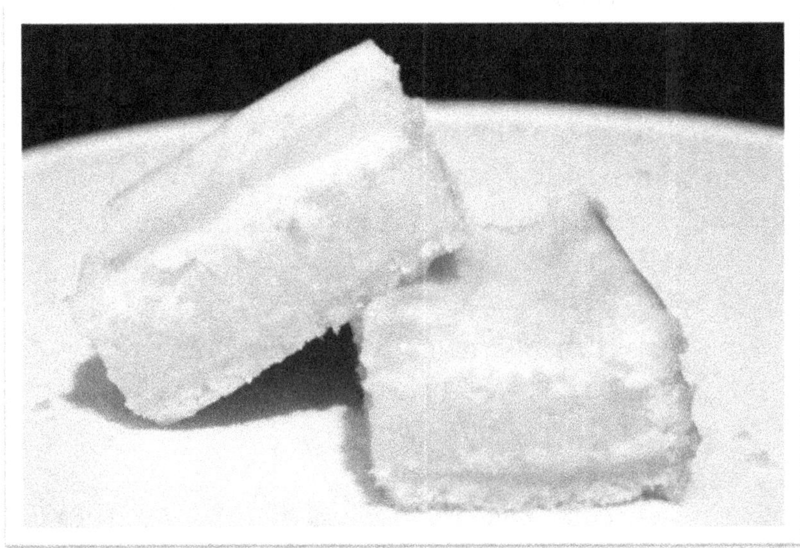

Yields: 12 servings
Total Time: 4 hours 10 minutes
Prep Time: 10 minutes
Cook Time: N/A

Ingredients

- ¼ cup melted coconut oil
- 4 tablespoons softened unsalted butter
- 4 ounces softened cream cheese
- 1 teaspoon fresh lemon juice
- 1 tablespoon fresh lemon zest
- Stevia
- Lemon extract

- Combine all ingredients in a bowl with a hand mixer.
- Blend until smooth and then pour into cupcake liners or molds.
- Freeze for at least 4 hours or until firm.
- Sprinkle with fresh lemon zest and serve.

Nutritional Information per Serving
Calories: 92;
Total Fat: 9.8 g;
Carbs: 0.8 g;
Dietary Fiber: 0 g;
Sugars: 0.5 g;
Protein: 0.9 g;
Cholesterol: 13 mg;
Sodium: 43 mg

Keto Peach Cobbler

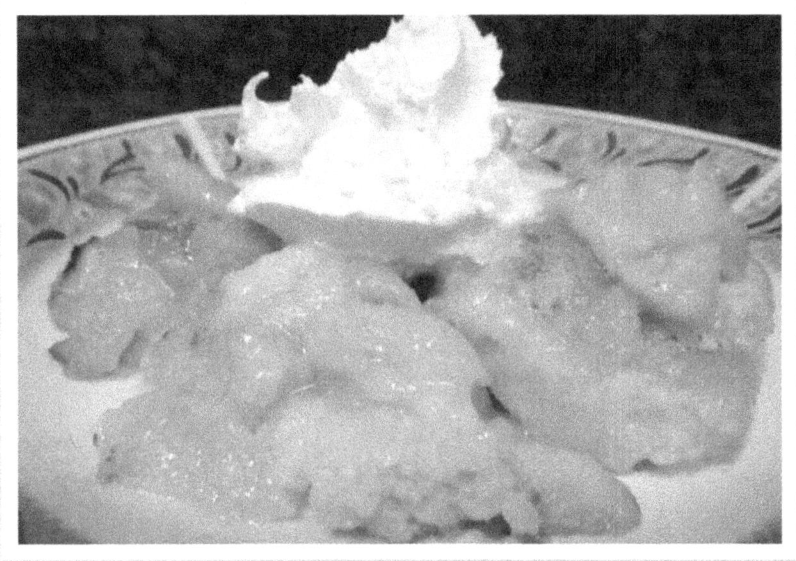

Yields: 1 serving
Total Time: 30 minutes
Prep Time: 10 minutes
Cook Time: 20 minutes

Ingredients

- 3 large ripe peaches, chopped
- 3 teaspoons coconut oil
- ½ cup almond flour
- 1 tablespoon cinnamon

- Add two cups of water to your instant pot and insert a trivet.
- In a bowl, mix together coconut oil, almond flour, and cinnamon until crumbles form.
- Add chopped peaches to a baking dish and sprinkle with almond flour crumbles. Cover with aluminum foil and place the dish on the trivet. Lock lid of the pot and cook on high for 20 minutes. Let pressure come down on its own. Serve warm.

Nutritional Information per Serving

Calories: 571;
Total Fat: 52.1 g;
Carbs: 10.5 g;
Dietary Fiber: 5.1 g;
Sugars: 1 g;
Protein: 23.4 g;
Cholesterol: 0 mg;
Sodium: 9,633 mg

Blissful Matcha-Pistachio Balls

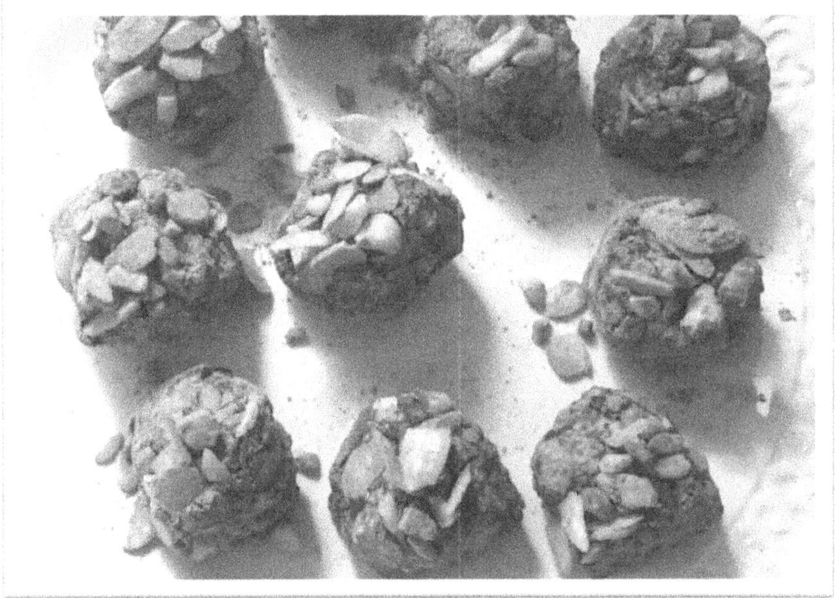

Yields: 4 servings
Total Time: 20 minutes
Prep Time: 5 minutes
Cook Time: N/A

Ingredients

- ½ cup shredded coconut, unsweetened
- 2 Medjool dates, pitted
- ¼ cup raw pistachios, shelled
- ¾ cup raw cashews
- 2 teaspoons matcha powder
- ¼ pistachios, chopped

- In a food processor, process together coconut, dates, cashews, and ¼ cup pistachios, and matcha powder until finely chopped.
- Roll into small balls and then roll the balls into the remaining chopped pistachios, pressing the pistachios firmly into the balls.
- Refrigerate the balls for about 15 minutes before serving.

Nutritional Information per Serving

Calories: 213;
Total Fat: 17.9 g;
Carbs: 9.4 g;
Dietary Fiber: 2.2 g;
Sugars: 2.3 g;
Protein: 5.4 g;
Cholesterol: 0 mg;
Sodium: 36 mg

Cashew Butter Fat Bombs

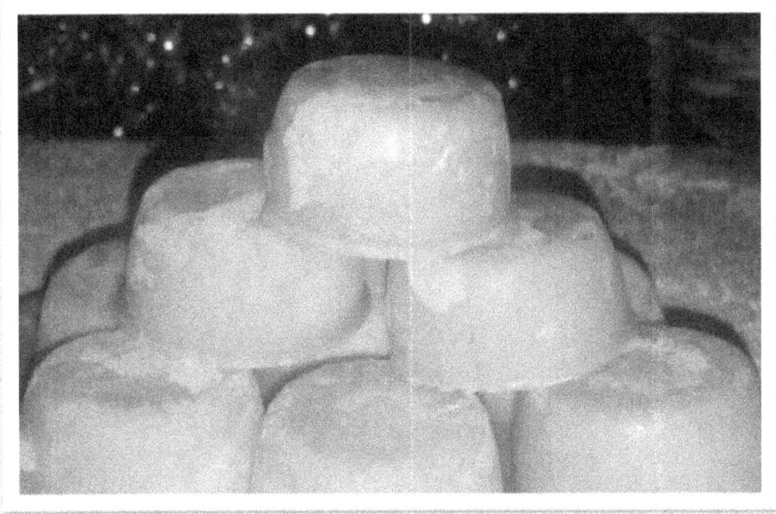

Yields: 12 Fat Bombs
Total Time: 25 minutes
Prep Time: 25 minutes
Cook Time: N/A

Ingredients

- 6 tablespoons cashew butter

- 6 tablespoons grass-fed butter

- ½ teaspoon liquid stevia

- 1 teaspoon vanilla extract

- 1 pinch of sea salt

- Prepare mini muffin tin by lining with liners. Set aside.
- In a microwave-safe bowl, mix grass-fed butter and cashew butter and then microwave for one minute or until melted. Stir in the remaining ingredients until well blended. Spoon the mixture into the prepared muffin tin and freeze for at least 10 minute or until firm. Enjoy!

Nutritional Information per Serving
Calories: 206;
Total Fat: 20 g;
Carbs: 5 g;
Dietary Fiber: 0.5 g;
Sugars: 1.6 g;
Protein: 2.1 g;
Cholesterol: 31 mg;
Sodium: 164 mg

Keto Cinnamon Roll Mousse

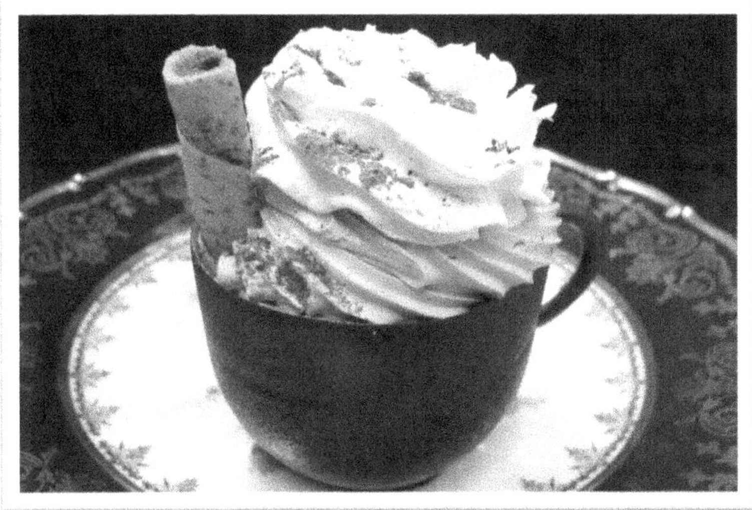

Yields: 4 servings
Total Time: 11 minutes
Prep Time: 10 minutes
Cook Time: 1 minute

Ingredients

- 2 tablespoons almond butter
- ½ cup cream cheese, softened
- ½ cup heavy whipping cream
- ¼ cup powdered Swerve
- ½ teaspoon sugar-free vanilla extract
- 1 teaspoon cinnamon

Drizzle

- 2 tablespoons coconut butter
- 1 tablespoon powdered Swerve
- 1 teaspoon virgin coconut oil

- Whisk together heavy cream and cream cheese until very smooth. Whisk in the remaining ingredients. In another bowl whisk together the drizzle ingredients until well combined. Microwave for about 10 seconds.
- Divide mouse among serving glasses and drizzle with the drizzle mixture. Sprinkle with cinnamon and serve. Enjoy!

Nutritional Information per Serving
Calories: 271;
Total Fat: 26.6 g;
Carbs: 5.7 g;
Dietary Fiber: 2.6 g;
Sugars: 1 g;
Protein: 4.7 g;
Cholesterol: 52 mg;
Sodium: 92 mg

Keto Almond Fudge Fat Bomb

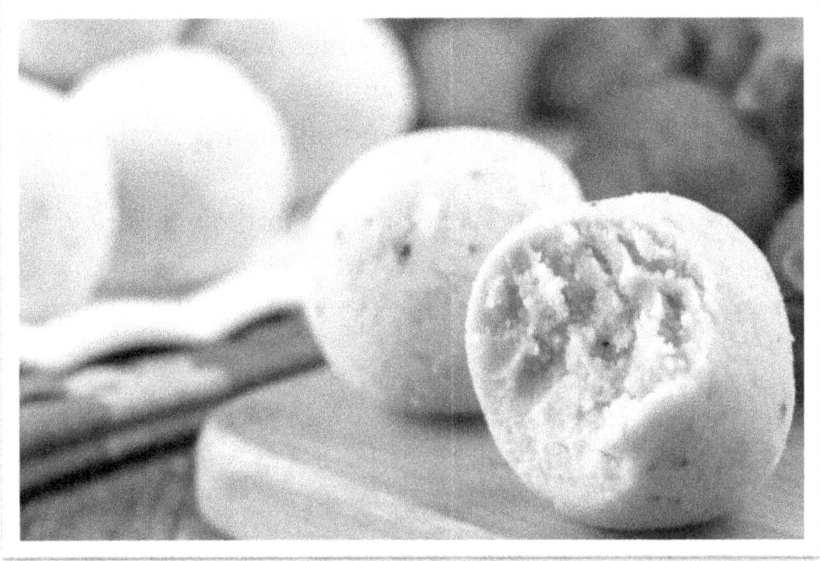

Yields: 24 Fat Bombs
Total Time: 1 hour 10 minutes
Prep Time: 10 minutes
Cook Time: N/A

Ingredients

- 2 tablespoons coconut oil

- ¼ cup butter

- ½ cup almond butter

- 1 tablespoon sugar-free maple syrup

- Melt coconut oil, butter, and almond butter for about 2 minutes in the microwave.
- Whisk until smooth and well combined.
- Whisk in maple syrup and then pour the mixture into muffin cups.
- Freeze for at least 1 hour or until firm. Enjoy!

Nutritional Information per Serving

Calories: 60;
Total Fat: 5 g;
Carbs: 1 g;
Dietary Fiber: 0 g;
Sugars: 0.4 g;
Protein: 1 g;
Cholesterol: 5 mg;
Sodium: 18 mg

Butter Onion Bacon Dessert

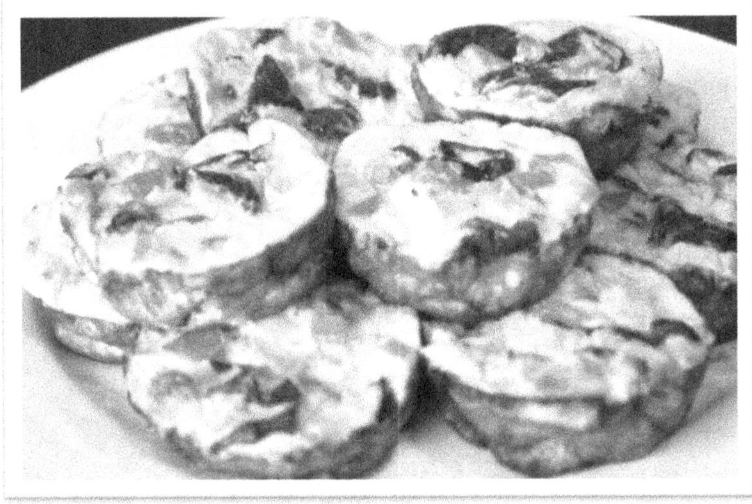

Yields: 12 Fat Bombs
Total Time: 20 minutes
Prep Time: 10 minutes
Cook Time: 10 minutes

Ingredients

- 4 strips bacon, sliced into small strips

- 9 tablespoons butter

- 90 g onion, diced

- ½ teaspoon pepper

- 2 teaspoons spicy brown mustard

- Add butter to a pan set over medium heat. Melt and cook in bacon for about 2 minutes. Add in onions and cook until bacon is crispy.

- Remove the pan from heat and let sit to cool for at least 5 minutes. Add in pepper and mustard until well blended. Divide the mixture among muffin cups and refrigerate until firm.

Nutritional Information per Serving
Calories: 92;
Total Fat: 10 g;
Carbs: 1 g;
Dietary Fiber: 0 g;
Sugars: 0 g;
Protein: 1 g;
Cholesterol: 23 mg;
Sodium: 151 mg

Spiced Low-Carb Coconut Milk Avocado Shake

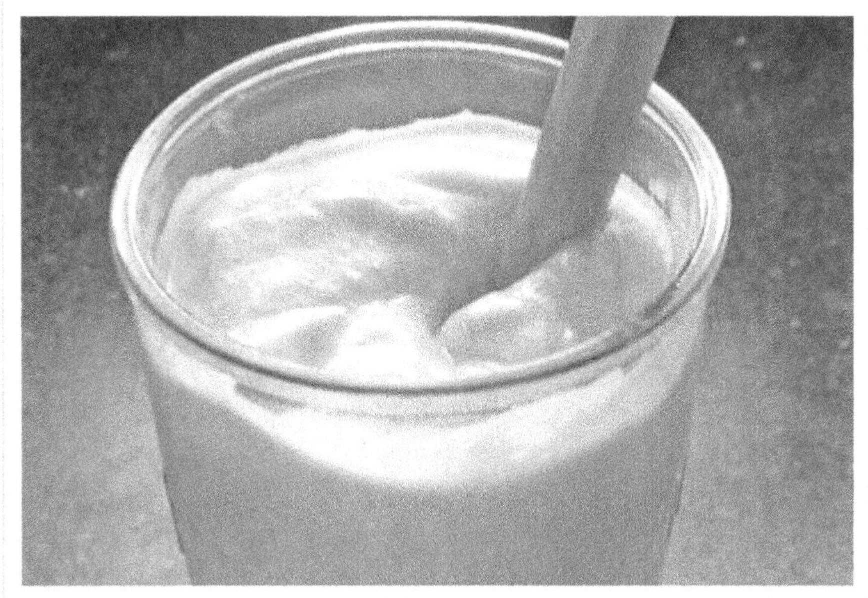

Yields: 2 servings
Prep Time: 5 minutes

Ingredients

- 2 tablespoons fresh lemon juice
- ½ avocado
- ¼ cup almond milk
- ¾ cup full-fat coconut milk
- 1 teaspoon fresh ginger, grated
- 1 scoop protein powder
- ½ teaspoon turmeric
- 1 cup crushed ice
- Stevia

Combine all ingredients in a blender and blend until very smooth. Enjoy!

Nutritional Information per Serving

Calories: 208;
Total Fat: 21 g;
Carbs: 5 g;
Dietary Fiber: 1.1 g;
Sugars: 2.2 g;
Protein: 11.9 g;
Cholesterol: 9 mg;
Sodium: 3 mg

Jalapeno Popper Fat Bombs

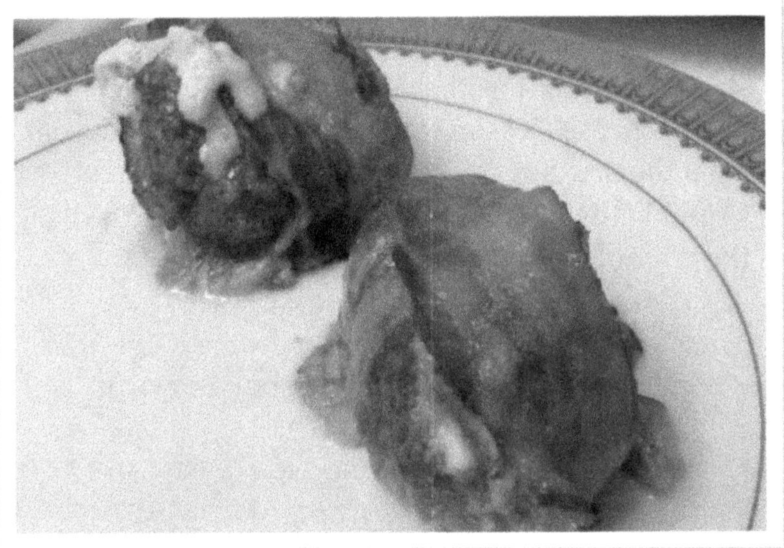

Yields: 10 Fat Bombs
Total Time: 20 minutes
Prep Time: 15 minutes
Cook Time: 5 minutes

Ingredients

- 3 slices bacon
- 2 jalapeno peppers, deseeded and diced
- ½ cup scallions, chopped
- 3 ounces cream cheese
- ¼ teaspoon garlic powder
- ¼ teaspoon onion powder
- ½ teaspoon dried parsley
- Salt & pepper, to taste

- In a skillet, fry bacon for about 5 minutes or until crisp. Transfer to paper towel to drain. Save bacon grease.
- In a bowl, mix together spices, scallions, bacon fat, and cream cheese. Season with salt and pepper and form balls from the mixture and set aside.
- Crumble the bacon and place in a bowl. Roll the balls into the crumbled bacon and serve.

Nutritional Information per Serving
Calories: 208;
Total Fat: 20.1 g;
Carbs: 1.2 g;
Dietary Fiber: 0 g;
Sugars: 1.1 g;
Protein: 4 g;
Cholesterol: 53 mg;
Sodium: 230 mg

Keto Cheese Roll-Ups

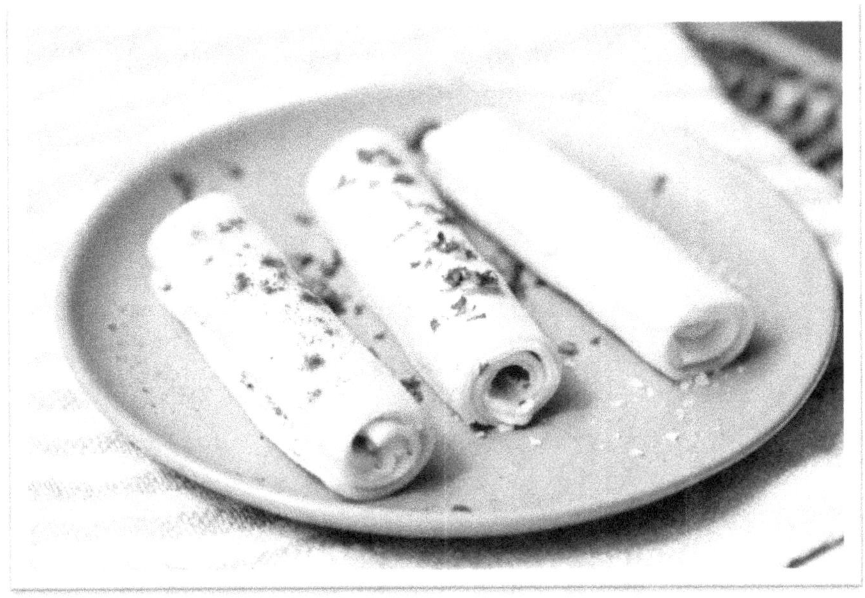

Yield: 1 Serving
Total Time: 10 Minutes
Prep Time: 10 Minutes
Cook Time: N/A

Ingredients

- 2 ounces sliced provolone, cheddar or edam cheese

- ½ ounce butter

- Place the cheese slices on a large cutting board.
- Slice butter with a cheese slicer or cut really thin pieces with a knife.
- Cover every cheese slice with butter and roll up. Serve as a snack.

Nutritional Information per Serving

Calories: 331;
Total Fat: 30 g;
Carbs: 2.4 g;
Dietary Fiber: 0.1 g;
Sugars: 1.1 g;
Protein: 13 g;
Cholesterol: 412 mg;
Sodium: 278 mg

Keto Biscuits & Gravy

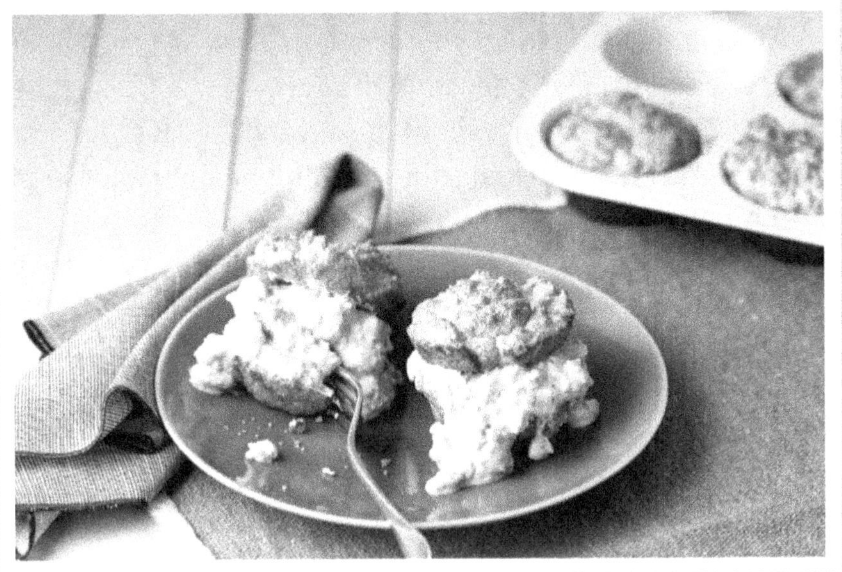

Yield: 2 Servings
Total Time: 25 Minutes
Prep Time: 10 Minutes
Cook Time: 15 Minutes

Ingredients

Biscuits

- 4 egg whites; 1 cup almond flour
- 1 teaspoon baking powder; ¼ teaspoon sea salt
- 2 tablespoons chilled butter
- 1 teaspoon garlic powder
- 1 teaspoon coconut oil spray

Gravy

- 1 cup coconut cream or cream cheese
- 10 ounces crumbled pork sausage
- 1 cup chicken or beef broth
- A pinch of sea salt; A pinch of black pepper

To make the Biscuits:

- Preheat the oven to 400°F (200°C). Coat your muffin pan or cookie sheet with coconut oil spray.
- Beat the egg whites in a bowl until very firm and fluffy.
- In another bowl, mix together the almond flour and baking powder.
- Mix in chilled butter and salt and then gently pour in the egg whites. Mix until well blended and spoon a dollop of the biscuit dough onto the prepared pan or sheet. Bake for about 11–15 minutes.

To make the Gravy:

- Add sausage to a large skillet set over medium heat and cook for about 5–6 minutes or until cooked through. Slowly stir in broth and cream cheese until the mixture comes to a gentle simmer. Lower heat and cook for about 2 minutes. Sprinkle with sea salt and pepper. Cut the biscuits into halves and serve two halves per plate with about a third cup of the gravy.

Nutritional Information per Serving
Calories: 358;
Total Fat: 33 g;
Carbs: 3.3 g;
Dietary Fiber: 0.3 g;
Sugars: 1.7 g;
Protein: 13 g;
Cholesterol: 218 mg;
Sodium: 387 mg

Low-Carb Crab Fat Bombs

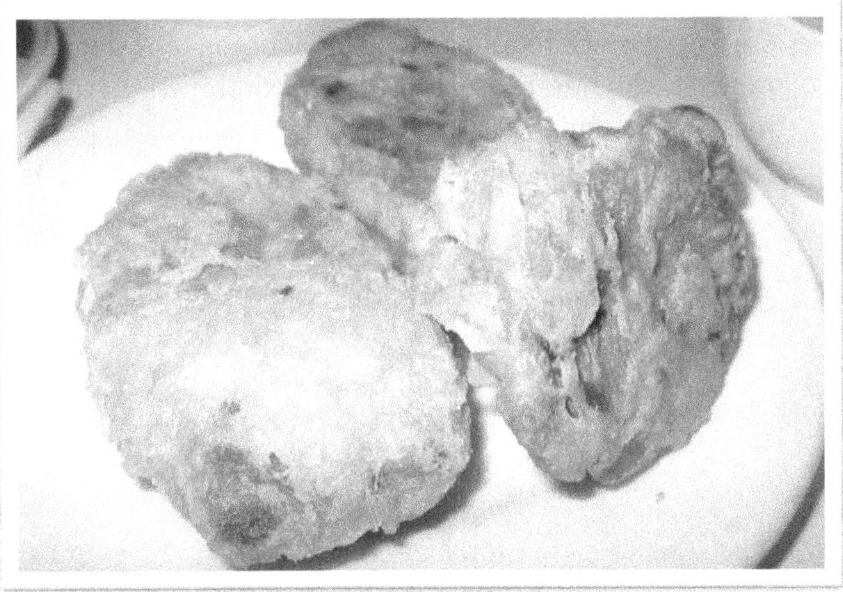

Yields: 24 Fat Bombs
Total Time: 15 minutes
Prep Time: 15 minutes
Cook Time: N/A

Ingredients

- 10 slices bacon
- ¾ cup mozzarella cheese, shredded
- 170 g crab
- 1 cup cream cheese
- 1 teaspoon onion powder
- 1 teaspoon garlic powder
- 1 teaspoon minced garlic
- Dash of salt and pepper

- In a bowl, mix together shredded mozzarella, cream cheese, canned crab meat, garlic, onion powder, garlic powder, salt, and pepper until well combined. Refrigerate for about 30 minutes.
- In a pan over medium-low heat, cook bacon until crispy. Chop into small pieces.
- Roll the crab-cheese mixture into small balls and then roll them into chopped bacon pieces. Enjoy!

Nutritional Information per Serving

Calories: 134;
Total Fat: 11.2 g;
Carbs: 2.9 g;
Dietary Fiber: 0.3 g;
Sugars: 1.6 g;
Protein: 10.5 g;
Cholesterol: 51 mg;
Sodium: 113 mg

Healthy Low-Carb Bagels

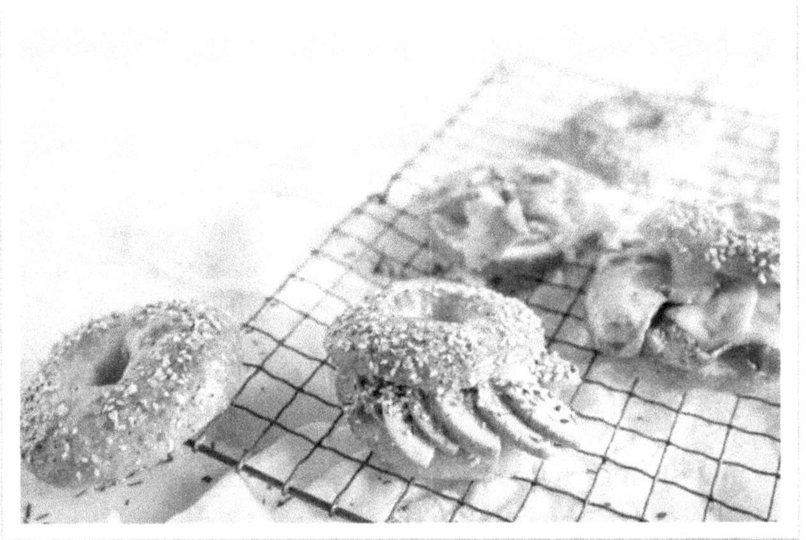

Yield: 3 Servings
Total Time: 31 Minutes
Prep Time: 15 Minutes
Cook Time: 16 Minutes

Ingredients

Bagels

- 7 ounces mozzarella cheese
- 1 ounce cream cheese
- 1½ cups almond flour
- 2 teaspoons baking powder
- 1 egg

Topping

- 2 teaspoons flaxseed
- 1 teaspoon sesame seeds
- ½ teaspoon sea salt
- ¼ teaspoon poppy seeds
- 1 egg

- Preheat the oven to 430°F (220°C). Prepare a baking tray by lining it with baking paper.
- Combine cream cheese and mozzarella in a microwave-safe bowl. Microwave on high for about a minute and then stir to combine well.
- In another bowl, mix together baking powder and almond flour until well blended. Whisk the egg and almond flour mix into the cheese mix to form a smooth dough. Divide dough into small portions and form bun shapes. Arrange on the prepared tray and press the centers of the buns with your hands to form bagel shapes. In a small bowl, whisk together the seasoning and the seeds until well combined.
- Add seasoning for the topping mix into a small bowl and give it a quick stir to combine.
- Beat the second egg into a small bowl until fluffy and light.
- Generously brush each bagel with the egg and sprinkle with the topping mixture. Bake in your preheated oven for about 15 minutes.

Nutritional Information per Serving
Calories: 493;
Total Fat: 41;
Carbs: 4.1 g;
Dietary Fiber: 1.1 g;
Sugars: 2.8 g;
Protein: 23 g;
Cholesterol: 387 mg;
Sodium: 391 mg

Keto BLT Baked Avocado Eggs

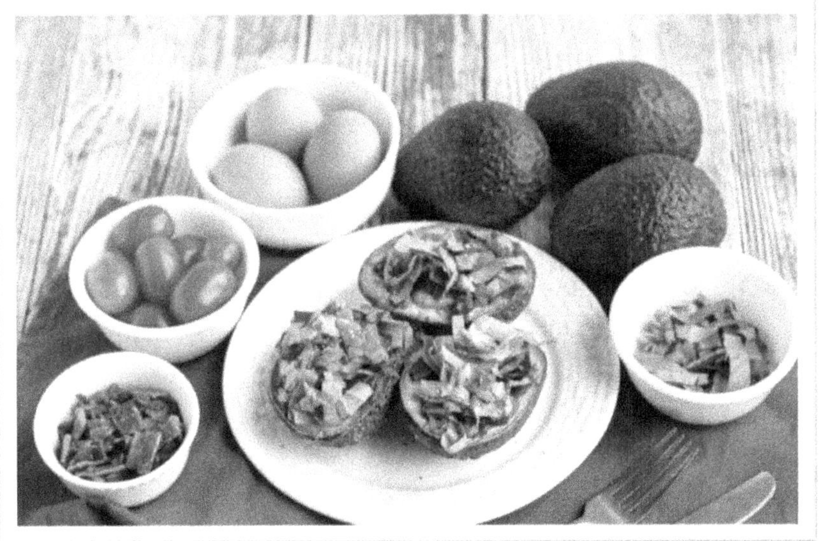

Yield: 4 Servings
Total Time: 35 Minutes
Prep Time: 15 Minutes
Cook Time: 20 Minutes

Ingredients

- 6 ounces bacon
- 2 avocados
- 4 eggs
- Salt and pepper, to taste
- 4 cherry tomatoes, quartered
- 1 ounce lettuce, shredded

- Add bacon to a skillet set over medium-high heat and fry until crispy. Remove from heat and cut into pieces. Set aside.
- Preheat your oven to 375 degrees.
- Slice the avocados into halves and remove the pits. Place the halves onto a baking pan and crack one egg into each half; season with sea salt and black pepper and then top with tomato slices and fried bacon.
- Bake in the preheated oven for about 15 to 20 minutes or until the eggs are cooked to your likeness. Serve the avocado eggs topped with the chopped lettuce.

Nutritional Information per Serving
Calories: 810;
Total Fat: 72 g;
Carbs: 17 g;
Dietary Fiber: 14.4 g;
Sugars: 3.2 g;
Protein: 26 g;
Cholesterol: 211 mg;
Sodium: 816 mg

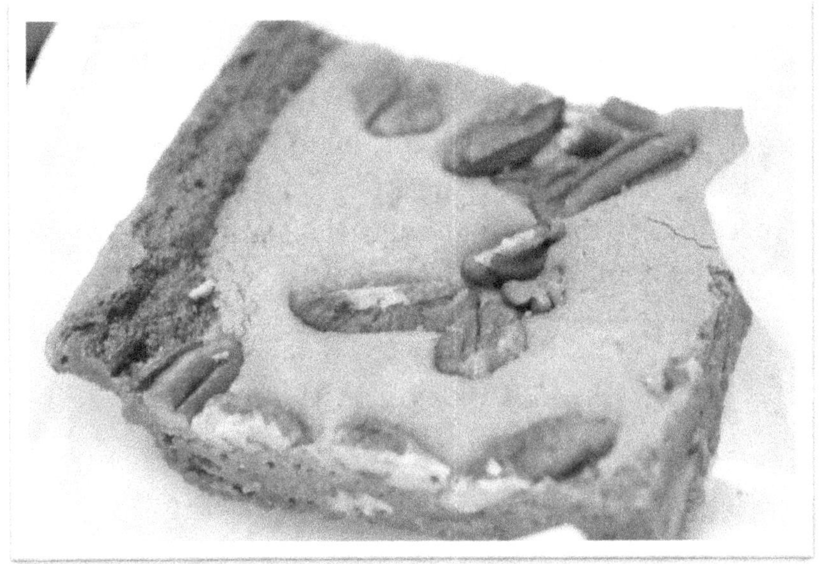

Yields: 10 Fudge Fat Bombs
Total Time: 4 hours 20 minutes
Prep Time: 20 minutes
Cooking Time: N/A

Ingredients

- ½ cup coconut oil
- 4 ounces food-grade cocoa butter
- 4 tablespoons unsweetened cocoa powder
- 1/3 cup heavy cream
- ½ cup pecans, roughly chopped
- 4 tablespoons erythritol/Swerve

- Melt coconut oil and cocoa butter in a double boiler. Whisk in cocoa powder until very smooth. Transfer to a blender. Add in the sweetener and blend until very smooth. Add in cream and continue blending for about 5 minutes.
- Arrange molds onto a sheet pan and fill each half with the pecans. Top each with the chocolate mixture and freeze for about 4 hours or until firm.

Nutritional Information per Serving
Calories: 494;
Total Fat: 53.1 g;
Carbs: 5.2 g;
Dietary Fiber: 2.2 g;
Sugars: 0.9 g;
Protein: 2.5 g;
Cholesterol: 11 mg;
Sodium: 4 mg

Keto Parmesan Croutons

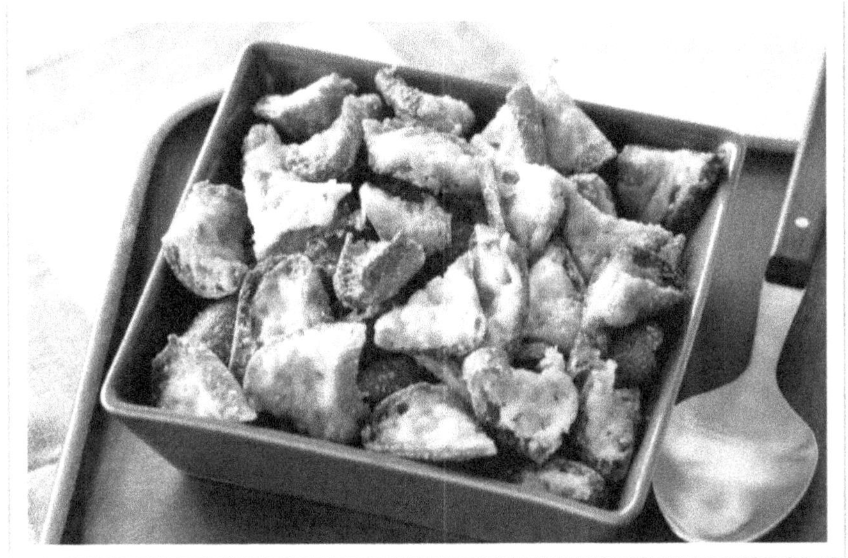

Yield: 3 Servings
Total Time: 55 Minutes
Prep Time: 15 Minutes
Cook Time: 40 Minutes

Ingredients

Parmesan Topping

- 4 ounces butter
- 3 ounces parmesan cheese, grated
- 1¼ cups almond flour
- 2 teaspoons baking powder
- 5 tablespoons ground psyllium husk
- 1 teaspoon sea salt
- 3 egg whites; 1¼ cups hot water
- 2 teaspoons cider vinegar

- Preheat the oven to 350 degrees. In a bowl, mix together all the dry ingredients until well combined.

- Bring a pan of water to a boil and then whisk into the dry ingredients along with egg whites and vinegar until you achieve a play-dough consistency.

- Form into 8 flat pieces of dough with moist hands. Remember that you need to allow a lot of room between the pieces as they will swell up to double their size as they are baked.

- Bake on lower rack of oven for about 40 minutes. Let cool for a few minutes. Split the bread pieces lengthwise and place both halves face-up on a sheet pan.

- Stir together the butter and parmesan cheese and spread on the halved bread. Raise the oven temperature to 450°F (220°C), or better yet, switch oven to a high broil. Pop bread pieces back in the oven for 5 minutes or until they have turned golden-brown. Watch continuously to avoid burning the topping.

- Enjoy whole as a snack, or split into smaller pieces, like in the picture above. Great with your favorite salad!

Nutritional Information per Serving
Calories: 272;
Total Fat: 24 g;
Carbs: 5.2 g;
Dietary Fiber: 4 g;
Sugars: 1.3 g;
Protein: 9 g;
Cholesterol: 210 mg;
Sodium: 512 mg

Low-Carb Italian Flaxseed Bread Crackers

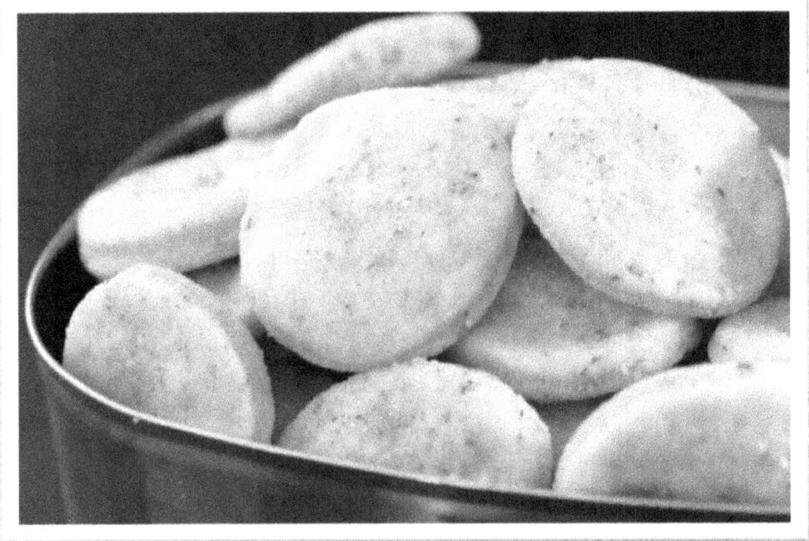

Yields: 4 servings
Total Time: 50 minutes
Prep Time: 15 minutes
Cook Time: 35 minutes

Ingredients

- 1 cup flaxseed meal
- ½ cup water
- 1 tablespoon Italian seasoning
- 2 teaspoons onion powder
- 1 tablespoon garlic powder
- 1 teaspoon salt

- Preheat oven to 400 degrees.
- In a bowl, mix together flaxseed meal and spices until well combined. Whisk in water and knead until the dough comes together. Transfer the dough onto a flat surface and roll it out to 0.3-cm thickness and then cut into small squares.
- Arrange the squares into a baking pan lined with parchment paper and bake for about 15 minutes. Carefully flip the bread cracker over and bake for another 20 minutes. Remove from oven and let cool before serving with garlic dip. Enjoy!

Nutritional Information per Serving
Calories: 151;
Total Fat: 12 g;
Carbs: 10 g;
Dietary Fiber: 10 g;
Sugars: 1 g;
Protein: 6 g;
Cholesterol: 9 mg;
Sodium: 240 mg

Low-Carb Pina Colada Fat Bombs

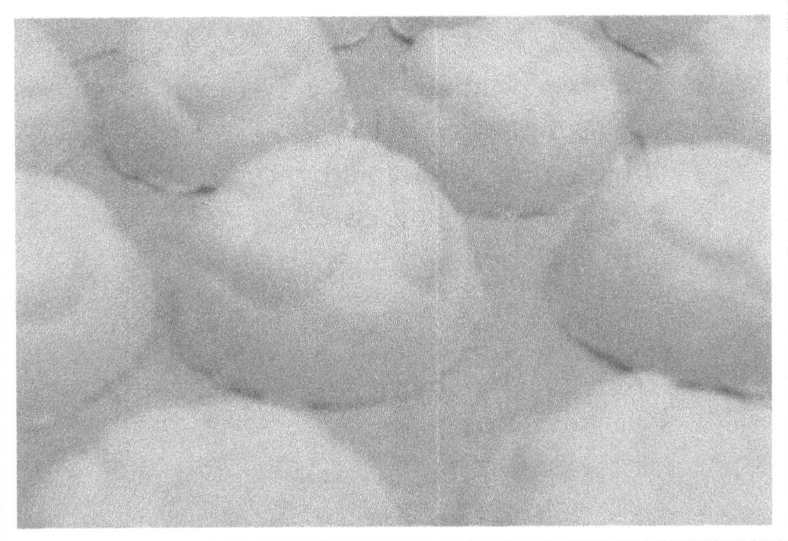

Yields: 16 Fat Bombs
Total Time: 1 hour 11 minutes
Prep Time: 10 minutes
Cook Time: 1 minute

Ingredients

- ½ cup coconut cream
- 2 teaspoons pineapple essence
- 3 teaspoons erythritol
- 2 scoops MCT Powder
- ½ cup boiling water
- 2 tablespoons gelatin
- 1 teaspoon rum extract

- Dissolve erythritol and gelatin in a jug of boiling water.
- Stir in pineapple essence and then let cool for at least 5 minutes.
- Stir in rum extract and coconut cream and then pour into silicon molds.
- Freeze for at least 1 hour. Enjoy!

Nutritional Information per Serving

Calories: 23;
Total Fat: 2.5;
Carbs: 0.4 g;
Dietary Fiber: 0.1 g;
Sugars: 0.2 g;
Protein: 2 g;
Cholesterol: 0 mg;
Sodium: 5 mg

Keto Lemon Poppy Seed Muffins Recipe

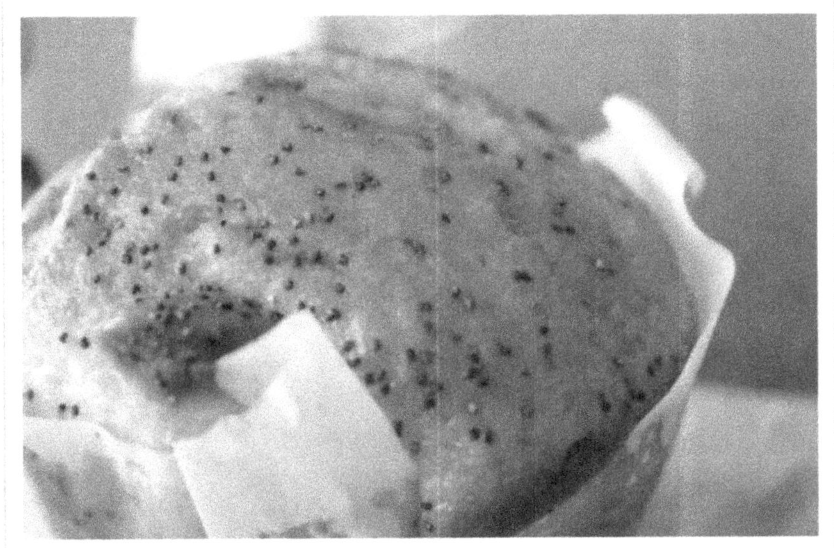

Yields: 12 servings
Prep Time: 10 minutes
Cook Time: 20 minutes
Total Time: 30 minutes

Ingredients

- 3 cups unblanched almond flour
- ½ cup grass fed butter, melted
- 3 free range eggs, whisked
- 2 ½ tablespoons poppy seeds
- 3 tablespoons (45 ml) lemon juice + zest of 1 lemon
- 1/3 cup stevia
- 1 teaspoon baking soda
- Dash of salt

- Start by setting your oven to 350 degrees F.
- Mix all the dry ingredients in a large mixing bowl and mix the butter and eggs in a separate bowl.
- Combine all the ingredients together then scoop the butter into your prepared muffin tin.
- Bake for about 16 minutes or until browned and an inserted toothpick comes out clean.
- Remove from oven and let cool.

Nutritional Information per Serving
Calories: 233;
Total Fat: 28 g;
Carbs: 6 g;
Dietary Fiber: 3 g;
Sugars: 1 g;
Protein: 7 g;
Cholesterol: 257 mg;
Sodium: 346 mg

Low-Carb Garlic Chia Bread Crackers

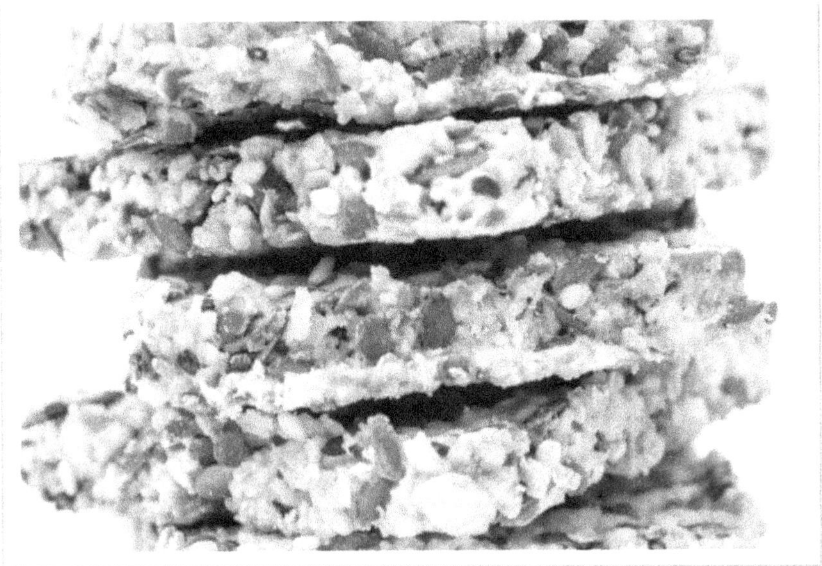

Yields: 4 servings
Total Time: 45 minutes
Prep Time: 15 minutes
Cook Time: 30 minutes

Ingredients

- 2 tablespoons chia seeds

- ½ cup chia or flax meal

- 1 tablespoon garlic powder

- 1 egg, whisked

- 1 teaspoon salt

- Preheat your oven to 300 degrees.
- In a bowl, mix together all ingredients until well blended. Place dough onto a flat surface and roll it out to 0.2-cm thickness and then cut into small squares.
- Arrange the squares into a baking pan lined with parchment paper and bake for about 30 minutes. Remove from oven and let cool before serving with garlic dip. Enjoy!

Nutritional Information per Serving
Calories: 123;
Total Fat: 9 g;
Carbs: 8 g;
Dietary Fiber: 5 g;
Sugars: 1 g;
Protein: 6 g;
Cholesterol: 104 mg;
Sodium: 211 mg

Low-Carb Bread Twists

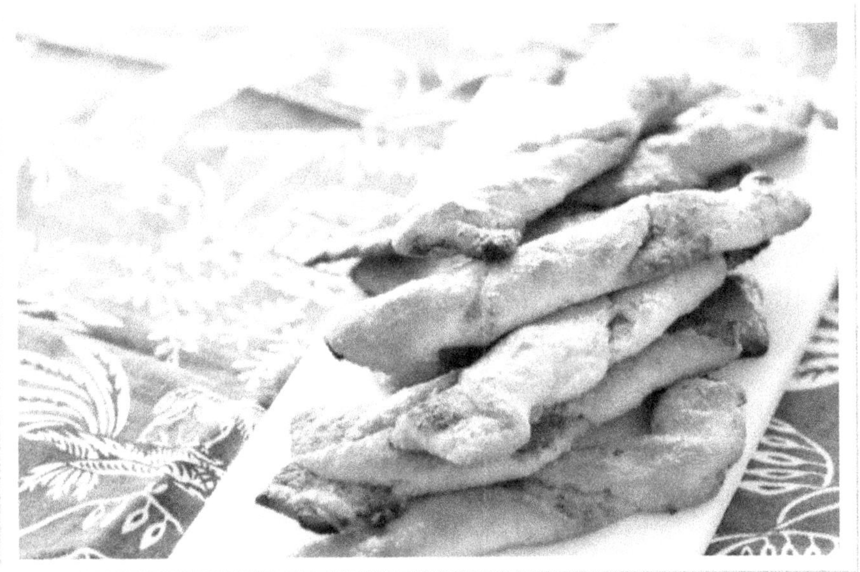

Yield: 2 Servings
Total Time: 40 Minutes
Prep Time: 20 Minutes
Cook Time: 20 Minutes

Ingredients

- ½ cup almond flour
- ¼ cup coconut flour
- ½ teaspoon salt
- 1 teaspoon baking powder
- 1 egg, beaten
- 2 ounces butter
- 6½ ounces shredded cheese, preferably mozzarella
- ¼ cup green pesto
- 1 egg, beaten, for brushing the top

- Preheat your oven to 350 degrees. In a bowl, mix together all the ingredients until well combined. Whisk in the egg and melted cheese and butter until well blended and smooth.
- Place dough onto a baking paper that has the same size as a rectangular cookie sheet. Use a rolling pin and make a rectangle, about 1/5-inch (5 mm) thick. Spread pesto on top and cut into 1-inch (2.5 cm) strips. Twist them and place on a baking sheet lined with parchment paper. Brush twists with the whisked egg.
- Bake in the oven for 15–20 minutes until they are golden-brown.

Nutritional Information per Serving

Calories: 194;
Total Fat: 17 g;
Carbs: 4.2 g;
Dietary Fiber: 2.1 g;
Sugars: 1.3 g;
Protein: 8 g;
Cholesterol: 112 mg;
Sodium: 705 mg

Simple and Quick Keto Muffins

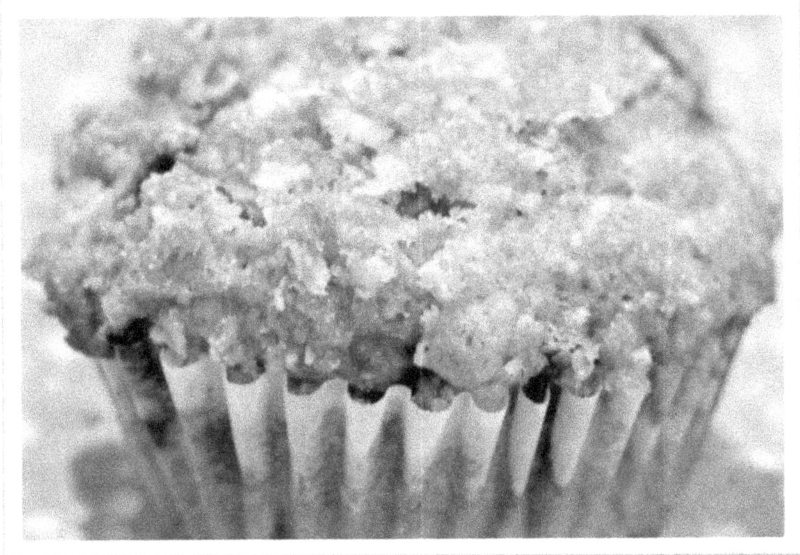

Yields: 4 servings
Total Time: 10 minutes
Prep Time: 5 minutes
Cook Time: 5 minutes

Ingredients

- 1 tablespoon coconut flour
- ½ tablespoon melted coconut oil
- 1 egg, beaten
- 1 tablespoon milk
- 1/8 teaspoon vanilla extract
- ½ teaspoon baking powder
- ¼ teaspoon honey
- 1 pinch of sea salt

- Preheat your oven to 350 degrees.
- In a bowl, mix together dry ingredients until well combined.
- In another bowl, whisk together wet ingredients until well blended. Gradually whisk in the dry ingredients until well blended. Transfer the batter to a ramekin and bake in the preheated oven for at least 15 minutes or golden-brown.
- Remove from oven and let cool before slicing to serve.

Nutritional Information per Serving
Calories: 200;
Total Fat: 12 g;
Carbs: 5 g;
Dietary Fiber: 2.5 g;
Sugars: 1 g;
Protein: 8 g;
Cholesterol: 198 mg;
Sodium: 413 mg

Chocolate & Pumpkin Protein Pudding

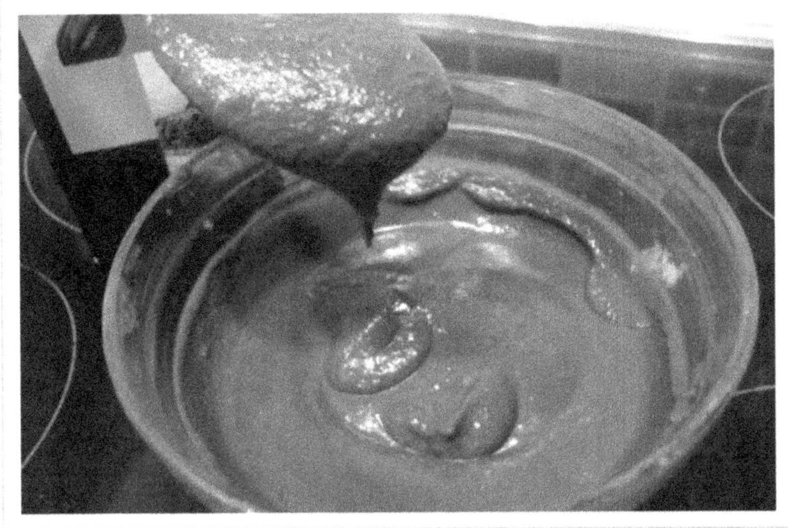

Yields: 6 servings
Total Time: 5 minutes
Prep Time: 5 minutes
Cook Time: N/A

Ingredients

- 1 cup almond milk
- 2 cups unsweetened pumpkin puree
- 3 tablespoons coconut oil
- ½ cup chocolate protein powder
- ¼ cup unsweetened cocoa powder
- ½ teaspoon ground cinnamon
- 1 teaspoon vanilla extract
- 1 teaspoon stevia

- In a blender, blend together pumpkin puree, coconut oil, protein powder, cinnamon, and vanilla until smooth.
- Add in half of the milk and blend until smooth.
- Add in the remaining milk and blend until very smooth.
- Refrigerate the shake for at least 2 hours before serving. Enjoy!

Nutritional Information per Serving

Calories: 234;
Total Fat: 15.1 g;
Carbs: 5.9 g;
Protein: 11.8 g;
Dietary Fiber: 1.8 g;
Sugars: 1.5 g;
Cholesterol: 1 mg;
Sodium: 15 mg

Cauliflower Breakfast Pizza

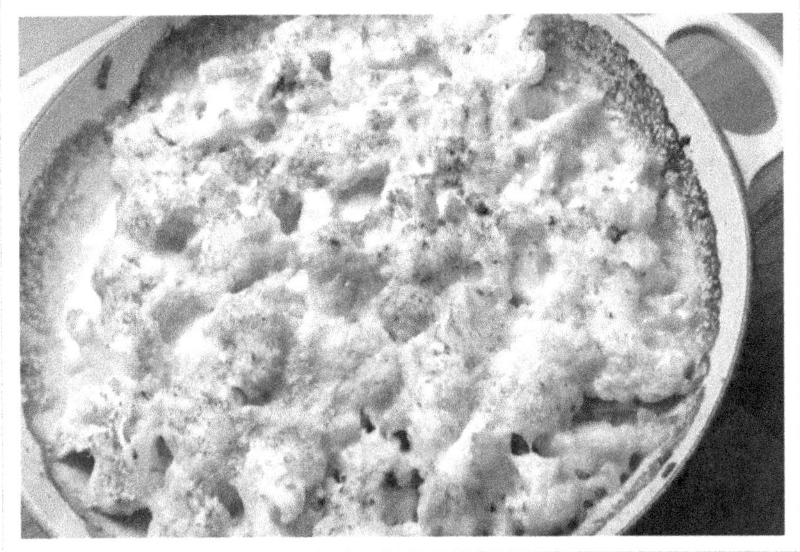

Yields: 2 servings
Prep Time 10 minutes
Cook Time 15 minutes
Total Time 25 minutes

Ingredients

- 2 cups riced cauliflower
- 4 free range eggs
- 2 tablespoons coconut flour
- ½ teaspoon kosher salt
- 1 tablespoon organic psyllium husk powder
- Toppings: Shredded cooked chicken, sliced avocado, halved cherry tomatoes crumbled goat cheese

- Start by setting your oven to 350 degrees F. Line your sheet pan with parchment paper.
- In a large glass bowl, combine all ingredients until evenly mixed. Let sit for 5 minutes for the dough to thicken and ingredients to marinate well.
- Spread the dough on the prepared sheet pan and use your hands to shape it into an even pizza crust. Bake for about 15 minutes, or until golden-brown.
- Remove from oven and top with toppings. Enjoy!

Nutritional Information per Serving

Calories: 454;
Total Fat: 31 g;
Carbs: 8.8 g;
Dietary Fiber 17.2 g;
Protein: 22 g;
Cholesterol: 1,325 mg;
Sodium: 188 mg

Tasty Keto Drop Biscuits

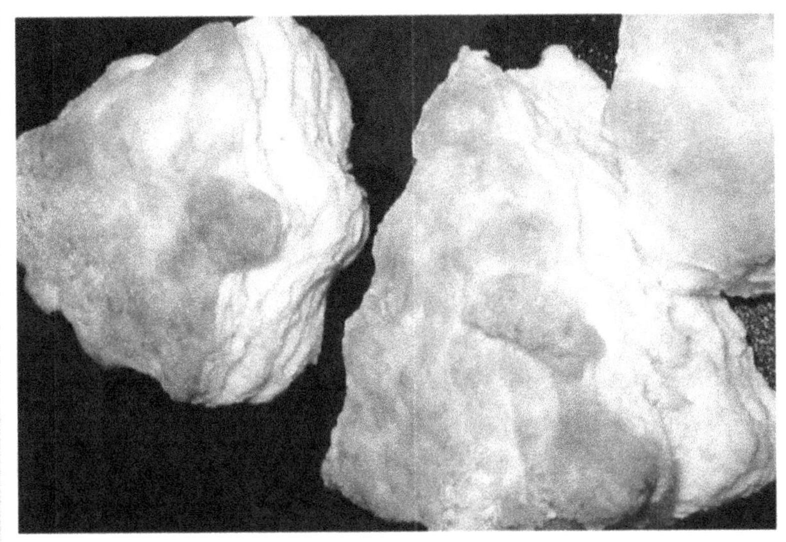

Yields: 3 servings
Prep Time: 10 minutes
Cook Time: 20 minutes
Total Time: 30 minutes

Ingredients

- 1 egg; 100 g coconut cream + 2 teaspoons apple cider vinegar, at room temp
- 2 tablespoons water
- 100 g almond flour
- 2 tablespoons coconut flour
- 2 tablespoons whey protein isolate or more almond flour
- 1 tablespoon apple cider vinegar
- 3 ½ teaspoons baking powder
- 1 tablespoon flaxseed meal
- 75 g golden flaxseed meal or psyllium husk, finely ground
- ½ teaspoon kosher salt
- 7 tablespoons ghee/coconut oil

- Preheat oven to 450 degrees F and line your baking tray with parchment paper or a baking mat.
- Whisk together the egg, coconut cream, water, and apple cider vinegar in a mixing bowl until very well combined and set aside.
- Stir the dry ingredients until well combined. You can use an electric mixer if you find this too cumbersome. Pour in the wet ingredients and continue pulsing. Add the ghee or coconut oil and pulse until well combined but sticky.
- Drop small rounds of dough using a serving spoon or tablespoon onto the prepared tray. Lightly brush with ghee and bake for about 15–20 minutes or until browned to desire.
- Remove from oven and let cool for 10 minutes before serving.

Nutritional Information per Serving

Calories: 290;
Total Fat: 30 g;
Carbs: 8 g;
Dietary Fiber 5 g;
Protein: 7 g;
Cholesterol: 74 mg;
Sodium: 455 mg

Chocolate Protein Fudge

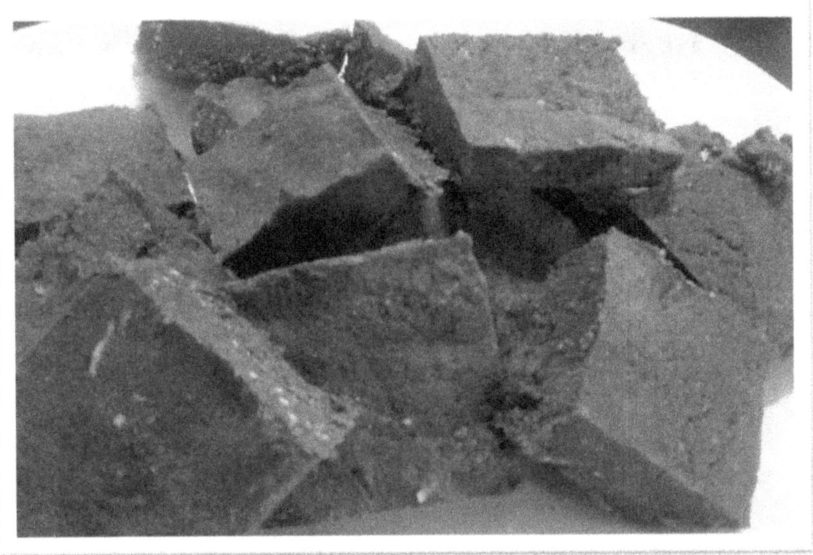

Yields: 6 servings
Total Time: 10 minutes + refrigerating time
Prep Time: 10 minutes
Cook Time: N/A

Ingredients

- 2 tablespoons almond butter
- ¼ cup dark chocolate chips
- 3 tablespoons coconut oil
- 2 tablespoons coconut flour
- 4 scoops protein powder
- 1 teaspoon cocoa powder
- 1 teaspoon vanilla
- 1 tablespoon stevia
- A pinch of sea salt

- In a bowl, mix together all ingredients (except a tablespoon of coconut oil and chocolate chips). Press the mixture into a glass container and refrigerate.
- In a pan over low heat, melt the remaining coconut oil and chocolate chips. Stir well and then pour over the fudge. Continue refrigerating for at least 30 minutes before slicing to serve.

Nutritional Information per Serving

Calories: 213;
Total Fat: 16.3 g;
Carbs: 7.2 g;
Protein: 10.2 g;
Dietary Fiber: 1.9 g;
Sugars: 3.2 g;
Cholesterol: 2 mg;
Sodium: 52 mg

Lime & Coconut Avocado Popsicles

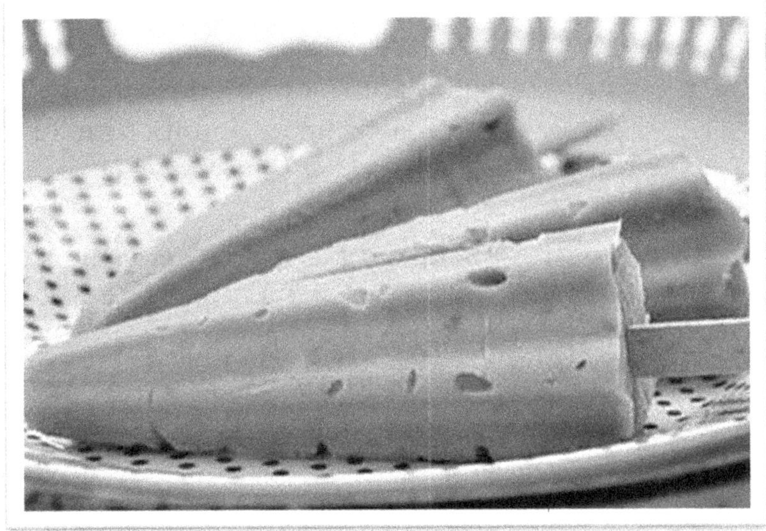

Yields: 3 servings
Total Time: 5 minutes + freezing time
Prep Time: 5 minutes
Cook Time: N/A

Ingredients

- 2 avocados

- 2 tablespoons lime juice

- 1 ½ cups coconut milk

- ¼ cup stevia

- In a blender, blend together all ingredients until smooth and creamy.
- Distribute the mixture into 6 Popsicle molds and the freeze for at least 2 hours or until firm. Enjoy!

Nutritional Information per Serving
Calories: 493;
Total Fat: 48.3 g;
Carbs: 10.9 g;
Protein: 8.4 g;
Dietary Fiber: 2.6 g;
Sugars: 6.5 g;
Cholesterol: 0 mg;
Sodium: 28 mg

Soft Rosemary-Infused Bagels

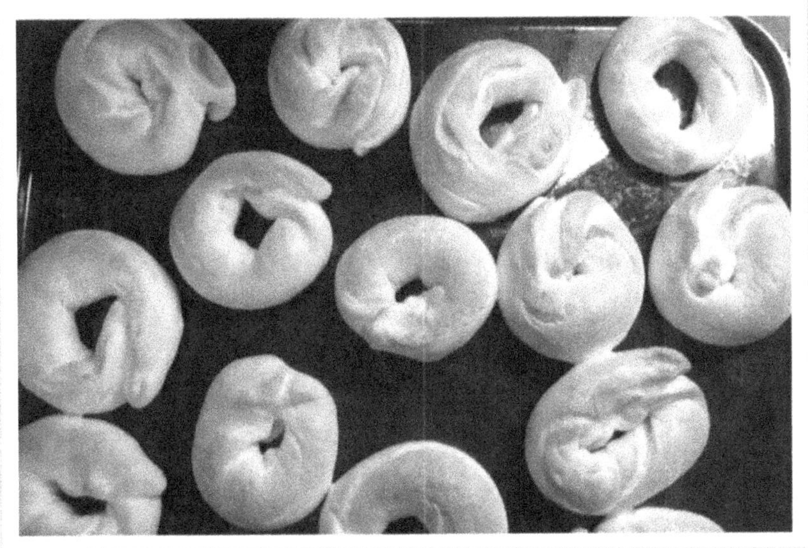

Yields: 4 servings
Total Time: 55 minutes
Prep Time: 5 minutes
Cook Time: 50 minutes

Ingredients

- 1 ½ cups coconut flour
- ¾ teaspoon baking soda
- ¾ teaspoon xanthan gum
- ¼ teaspoon salt
- 3 tablespoons ground flaxseed
- 1 egg; 3 egg whites
- ½ cup warm water
- 1 tablespoon fresh rosemary, finely chopped
- Avocado oil

- Set your oven to 250 degrees F.
- Mix all the dry ingredients (apart from ground flaxseed) in a bowl.
- Whisk eggs and warm water in a separate bowl. Stir in ground flaxseed until there are no clumps.
- Add the egg mixture to the dry ingredients and knead until the dough becomes elastic. Shape it into a bagel and coat with avocado oil.
- Press dough into a silicon mold and lightly press the chopped rosemary on top.
- Bake in the heated oven for 40 to 50 minutes or until browned to desire.

Nutritional Information per Serving
Calories: 285;
Total Fat: 22.5 g;
Carbs: 12 g;
Dietary Fiber 7.5 g;
Protein: 13 g;
Cholesterol: 46 mg;
Sodium: 82.5 mg

Fluffy Turmeric Veggie Buns

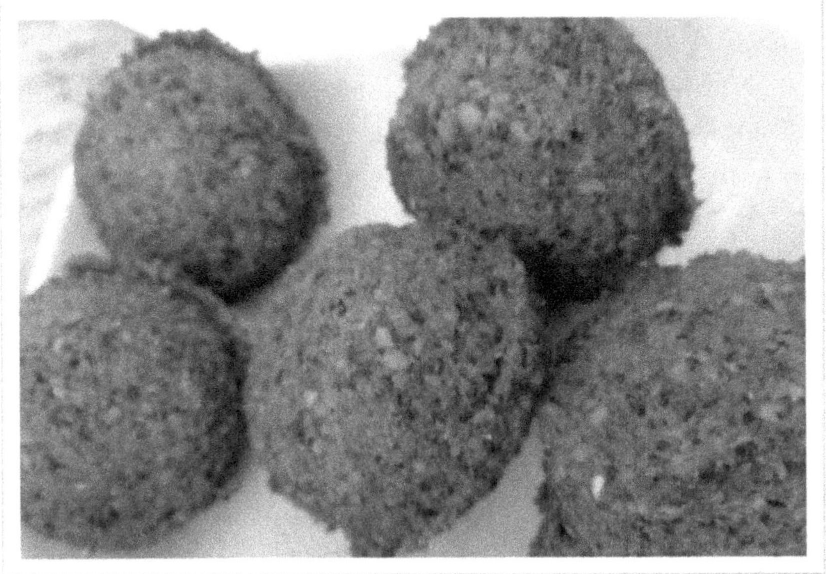

Yields: 4 servings
Total Time: 60 minutes
Prep Time: 30 minutes
Cook Time: 30 minutes

Ingredients

- 2 cups fresh riced cauliflower
- 2 free-range eggs
- 2 tablespoons almond flour
- 2 tablespoons olive oil
- ¼ teaspoon ground turmeric
- Kosher salt and freshly ground pepper, to taste

- Preheat your oven to 400 degrees and line a baking sheet with parchment paper or use a non-stick one.
- Microwave the cauliflower for 3 minutes then set aside to cool slightly. Transfer to a cheesecloth and squeeze out the water until dry then set aside in a large mixing bowl. Whisk in the eggs, oil, salt, pepper, and turmeric.
- You can use your hands at this point. Once mixed well, form 6 buns and arrange them on the prepared sheet and bake for about half an hour or until golden.
- Serve hot!

Nutritional Information per Serving

Calories: 221;
Total Fat: 9.3 g;
Carbs: 8 g;
Dietary Fiber 6 g;
Protein: 8 g;
Cholesterol: 34 mg;
Sodium: 79 mg

Almond Flour Italian Crackers

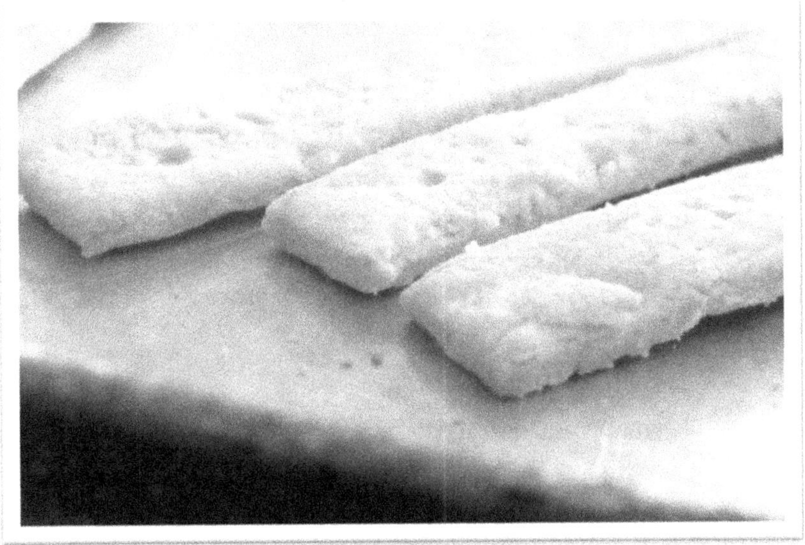

Yields: 3 servings
Prep Time: 5 minutes
Cook Time: 15 minutes
Total Time: 20 minutes

Ingredients

- 1 ½ cups almond flour
- 1 egg
- 2 tablespoons olive oil
- ¾ teaspoon salt
- ¼ teaspoon basil
- ½ teaspoon thyme
- ¼ teaspoon oregano
- ½ teaspoon onion powder
- ¼ teaspoon garlic powder

- Preheat your oven to 350 degrees F and line a baking tray with parchment paper.
- Combine all the ingredients in a large mixing bowl. Shape the dough into a long rectangular or circular log and cut into thin slices.
- Arrange the slices on the baking tray. It makes about 20–30 crackers. Bake for 10–12 minutes or until browned to desire.

Nutritional Information per Serving

Calories: 111;
Total Fat: 4 g;
Carbs: 9 g;
Dietary Fiber 4 g;
Sugars: 4 g;
Protein: 7 g;
Cholesterol: 49 mg;
Sodium: 211 mg

Chocolate Peanut Butter Milkshake

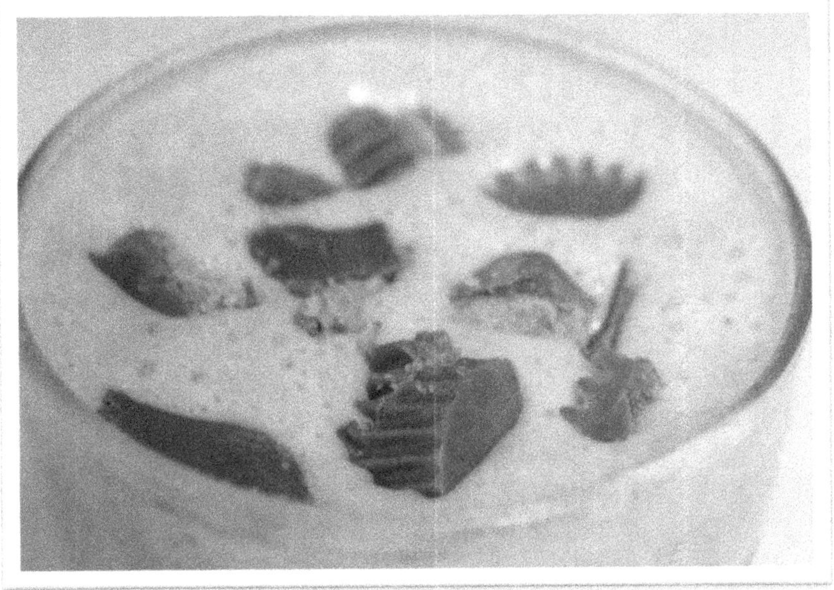

Yields: 1 serving
Total Time: 5 minutes
Prep Time: 5 minutes
Cook Time: N/A

Ingredients

- 1 tablespoon natural peanut butter
- 1 tablespoon unsweetened cocoa powder
- 1 cup unsweetened coconut milk
- Pinch of sea salt
- 1 teaspoon liquid stevia
- 1 scoop protein powder

Blend all ingredients together until smooth. Enjoy!

Nutritional Information per Serving

Calories: 664;
Total Fat: 66 g;
Carbs: 19.2 g;
Dietary Fiber: 8.1 g;
Sugars: 9.1 g;
Protein: 31.6 g;
Cholesterol: 0 mg;
Sodium: 274 mg

Cheese & Fruit-Stuffed Panini

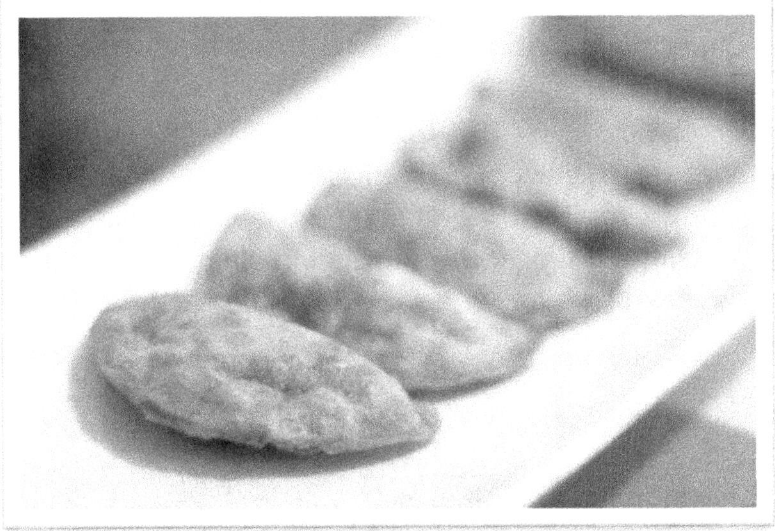

Yields: 10 Sandwiches
Prep Time: 10 minutes
Cook Time: 30 minutes
Total Time: 40 minutes

Ingredients

- Low-carb flatbread (10 slices)
- 2 tablespoons Dijon mustard
- 2 tablespoons mayonnaise
- 250 g aged ham
- 120 g brie, thinly sliced
- 1 green apple, very thinly sliced
- Oil or melted butter for brushing

- Start by preheating your Panini maker.
- Cut through the center of each slice of bread to get two very flat and thin slices.
- Combine mustard and mayonnaise in a small bowl and spread one side of all the slices with the combo. And form sandwiches with the cheese and ham. Brush the outer parts of the sandwiches with the melted butter and put in the Panini maker leaving it grill until golden.

Nutritional Information per Serving
Calories: 288;
Total Fat: 12 g;
Carbs: 15.5 g;
Dietary Fiber 7.1 g;
Protein: 13.6 g;
Cholesterol: 217 mg;
Sodium: 329 mg

Healthy Grain-Free Bagels

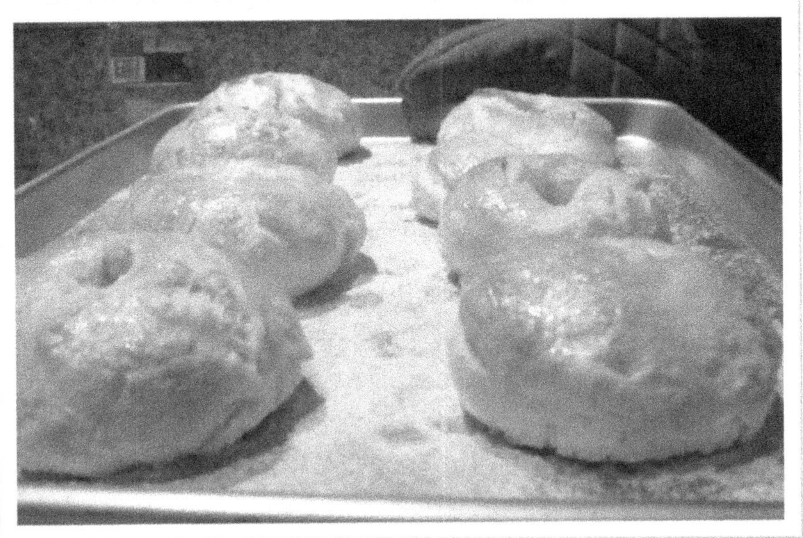

Yields: 6 Bagels
Total Time: 30 minutes
Prep Time: 10 minutes
Cook Time: 20 minutes

Ingredients

- ¼ cup sour cream

- 1 ½ cups almond flour

- 3 eggs

- Preheat your oven to 350 degrees. Grease five wells in a donut pan. Set aside.
- Beat eggs until creamy and light. Stir in sour cream until very smooth. Mix in almond flour until well combined. Spread the batter into the donut molds. Bake for about 20 minutes. Let cook and slice to serve. Best served toasted with sour cream or butter.

Nutritional Information per Serving

Calories: 225;
Total Fat: 17.2 g;
Carbs: 7.9 g;
Dietary Fiber 1.2 g;
Protein: 15.6 g;
Cholesterol: 199 mg;
Sodium: 231 mg

Superfood Keto Shake

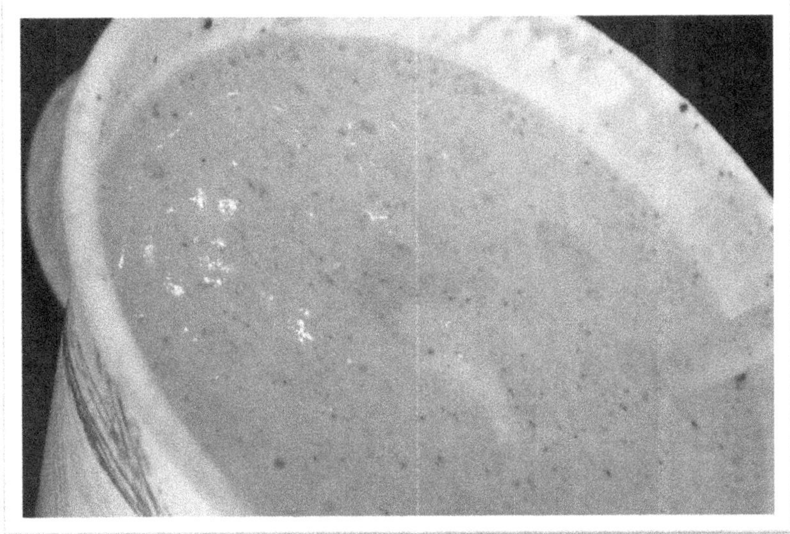

Yields: 2 servings
Prep Time: 5 minutes

Ingredients

- 1 tablespoon peanut butter
- 1 tablespoon MCT Oil
- 1 cup unsweetened almond milk
- 2 teaspoons acai powder
- 2 teaspoons maca powder
- 2 teaspoons chia seeds
- 1 handful ice

In a blender, blend together all ingredients until very smooth. Enjoy!

Nutritional Information per Serving
Calories: 287;
Total Fat: 28.2 g;
Carbs: 6.5 g;
Dietary Fiber: 1.6; g;
Sugars: 1.8 g;
Protein: 11.1 g;
Cholesterol: 0 mg;
Sodium: 113 mg

Healthy Mocha Ice Bombs

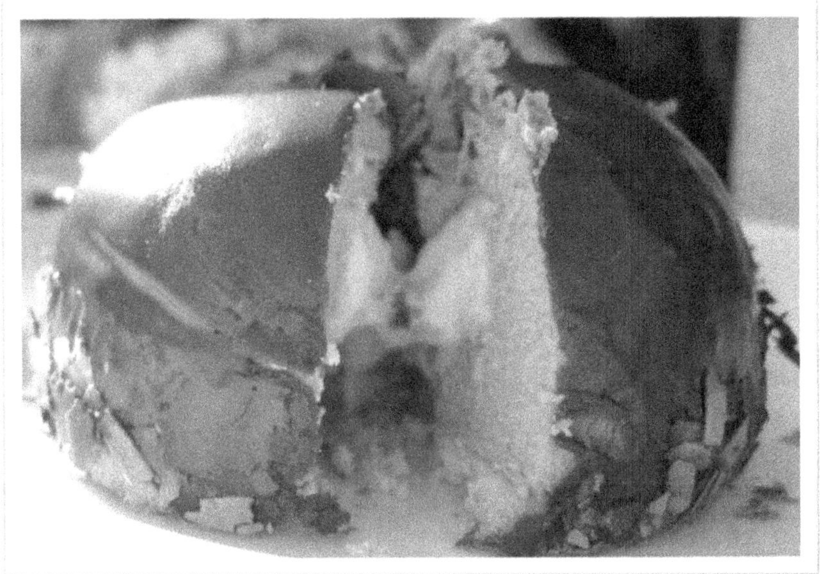

Yields: 20 Fat Bombs
Total Time: 1 hour 10 minutes
Prep Time: 10 minutes
Cook Time: N/A

Ingredients

- 240 g cream cheese
- 60 ml strong coffee, chilled
- 2 tablespoons cocoa powder
- 4 tablespoons powdered sweetener

Chocolate Coating

- 28 g cocoa butter, melted
- 70 g dark chocolate, melted

- In a bowl, whisk together melted cocoa butter and chocolate until well blended. Set aside.
- In a food processor, pulse together cocoa powder, cream cheese, coffee, and sweetener until very smooth. Roll the mixture into bite-sized balls and then dip them into the cocoa butter mixture and arrange them on a baking tray lined with baking paper. Refrigerate for at least 1 hour before serving.

Nutritional Information per Serving

Calories: 127;
Total Fat: 12.9 g;
Carbs: 2.2 g;
Dietary Fiber: 0.7 g;
Sugars: 1.1 g;
Protein: 1.9 g;
Cholesterol: 22 mg;
Sodium: 94 mg

We humans have varying opinions on everything by our very nature, but the one topic we agree on is the desire of health in the mind, body, and soul. We want a life without stress, a healthy weight, young, glowing skin, eight hours of sleep, and a life of complete Zen.

If I were to tell you that the keto diet will help you achieve all the above, that would be a lie. But the one thing I can tell you for sure, from my own experience, is that it will help you reboot your system, boost your energy levels, lose weight, prevent and reduce symptoms of chronic illnesses, and allow you to live a healthy life while enjoying very tasty and filling recipes.

Not much of a baker or dessert connoisseur? This is the perfect healthy dessert book for you! I am not one either, but the one thing that's true, as I mentioned at the beginning of the book, is that I love, love, love desserts! You will find that all the recipes are super simple, take very little time, don't require crazy ingredients, and the most important thing—they will blow your taste buds off!

Now you can officially start hosting brunches that feature desserts or dinners where you save the best for last! Let us spread the word on how possible it is to eat dessert and lose weight. Food is meant to nourish us and make us healthy, not leave us feeling like failures simply because we equate each bite to the calories we are going to gain.

Food is one of the things that bring people together. This book will help you cook with more soul, and the aromas floating from your kitchen will create some of the best memories for you and your friends and family.

I am so happy to have shared this knowledge that took me years to gain, but that changed my life, and I hope that you, too, will share this book far and wide to help as many people as possible. We are together in this! Forever in my mind!

Congratulations on going through this book and using the recipes! I hope this was a fun, tasty, and educative experience and that you are going to be making these recipes on a regular basis. I am positive that this simple recipe book will finally retire you from what has seemingly been a very long career in dieting.

You have gained a wealth of knowledge; use it well and share it widely with your friends and family to help out someone who is also stuck like you and I were. Embrace the keto diet and follow it daily, and weight is no longer going to be one of your problems.

These desserts are a great way for you to feed your kids tasty treats without having to worry that it could have negative effects on them, and you will also be teaching them healthy habits that they are going to carry into adulthood.

Feel free to switch up the recipes to your favorite specifications or in a way that works even more perfect for you. Get creative and come up with new recipes and remember to share them with me. As you prepare these recipes, you will be connecting with so many more people who are using this book. Also, feel free to suggest topics that you would want me to cover in the next book.

All the best as you embark on this beautiful health journey!

Jessica Logan